"Cheryl L. Woods Giscombé is a guru, and this guide is long overdue. She is the pioneer of the Superwoman Schema, and her research is legendary. She is one of the reasons why I chose this as one of my favorite interests. This guide promises to illuminate how to better ourselves and liberate us all from feeling like the world is on our shoulders and is ours to fix."

> —**C. Nicole Swiner, MD**, family doctor, speaker, and
> author of *How to Avoid the Superwoman Complex* and
> *The Superwoman Complex*

"Absolutely brilliant and empowering! I literally felt lighter and more joyful after reading this book and putting the strategies immediately into practice. I am excited and truly grateful to have such an important work to share with my clients, and to wholeheartedly recommend to all. The insights bring us into the unique experience of the Black woman in a way that has the power to inform and serve us all."

> —**Keitra M. Robinson, JD, CPEC**, founder of Justinspire
> Legends International Coaching and Consulting, and
> author of *Life Re-Imagined*

"This book is a love letter to Black women who struggle with the need to be strong, stoic, invulnerable, relentlessly resilient, and to put everyone else's needs before their own. In this thoughtful and inspirational guide, Cheryl Giscombé weaves real-world narratives of stress, strength, and their impact on Black women's health with loving, practical strategies of how Black women can better cope—and live happier and fuller lives."

> —**Tené T. Lewis, PhD, FAHA, FABMR, FAPA**,
> professor of epidemiology in the Rollins School of Public
> Health at Emory University

"*The Black Woman's Guide to Coping with Stress* offers Black women everywhere a chance to heal, transform, and evolve through mindful living and self-reflection. This book is a representation of many of us and offers practical, grounded advice to overcome generational ways of being that have left us sick, depleted, and fatigued. The mindfulness practices shared are a portal for liberation for those of us who have been wearing the 'superwoman' cape for far too long."

—**Dora Kamau, BScRPN**, headspace mindfulness meditation teacher

The Voices for Change Series

Mental health equity is a social justice issue. Written by leaders in psychology, sociology, gender, and ethnic studies, the New Harbinger *Voices for Change* series gives voice to the experience of marginalized people, and offers culturally informed, evidence-based strategies to help you cope with a broad range of social inequities that impact well-being and quality of life.

As research has shown us, social oppression can lead to mental health issues such as anxiety, depression, trauma, lowered self-esteem, and self-harm. These books provide practical tools based in proven-effective therapeutic methods to help you cultivate self-awareness, unlearn internalized negative messages, and build the inner resources you need to thrive.

For a complete list of books in
the *Voices for Change* series,
visit newharbinger.com

The Black Woman's Guide to Coping with Stress

Mindfulness & Self-Compassion Skills to Create a Life of Joy & Well-Being

CHERYL L. WOODS GISCOMBÉ, PHD, RN

New Harbinger Publications, Inc.

Publisher's Note

NEW HARBINGER PUBLICATIONS is a registered trademark of New Harbinger Publications, Inc.

New Harbinger Publications is an employee-owned company.

Distributed in Canada by Raincoast Books

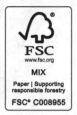

Copyright © 2024 by Cheryl L. Woods Giscombé
New Harbinger Publications, Inc.
5720 Shattuck Avenue
Oakland, CA 94609
www.newharbinger.com

Cover design by Sara Christian

Interior design by Tracy Marie Carlson

Acquired by Tesilya Hanauer

Edited by Karen Schader

Library of Congress Cataloging-in-Publication Data on file

Printed in the United States of America

26   25   24

10   9   8   7   6   5   4   3   2   1   First Printing

Contents

Foreword

All humans need healing, at times.

And even though, for each of us, our precise needs are not the same, we do all need to find the pathways to healing that are supportive for us.

For people who identify as Black women, the vulnerabilities that every human being faces in a life of any length are multiplied, indeed compounded, by other facts that arise in our cultures and communities and lead to what has been called, aptly, "surplus suffering" (Powell 2003). These facts—racism, sexism, and their associated politics and policies—are what intersect and lead to interlocking, systemic biases against women of color, and their follow-on disadvantaging consequences.

Add to these facts the realities of other forms of disadvantage and bias—disability, immigration status, religious minoritization, and so forth—and the myriad and unique ways that *each and every Black woman* has encountered harm in the social world, and suffered because of it, become, if not entirely clear, at least somewhat cognizable.

It is not possible to fully articulate the challenges that Black women face in the effort to, as my grandmother used to say, "make a way out of no way," each day in the particular circumstances in which she finds herself.

Of these realities, given that you are reading these words, you already know at least something. Grounded in your own experience, you know something unique and important about how race and class and religion and gender or sexuality have led to particular kinds of joy and meaning, on the one hand, but also, to particular kinds of blues and pain.

Because we know that these unique ways of suffering are the reality of Black women's lives, we fail to at least try to identify and work to alleviate the stress and pain that they cause at our collective moral peril. And as Black women, we ourselves must try even harder to find ways of understanding and alleviating our pain, because, indeed, not only our lives, but the lives of so many others—our families, workplaces, and political moments that depend on us for their survival—are imperiled.

The great gift of this book is that Dr. Giscombé does so much more than merely try. Drawing on her unique combination of personal experience, research-based excellence, and immersion in the techniques and studies of skilled, compassionate care, Dr. Giscombé gives us words and concepts to help us better describe what we are feeling and going through.

And she provides a range of traditionally-inspired, original practices to assist us in doing the part of the work of healing that is ours alone to do.

There is no question that the work that we can each personally do is not *all* of what must be done—we still need systemic change, a politics of dignity and liberation that opens doors for us, and for everyone. And so much more.

Nevertheless, for each of us—for you, facing whatever illness or setback, great or small that led you to pick up this book; for me, facing my own—the pages that we now behold offer a bridge of support, over which we can cross as we move in the direction of healing that we all seek.

So, join with me in doing the healing work that this wonderful book invites us to do.

Let's allow this book to be a bridge, or a window, or a doorway into the particular path toward healing that is yours alone to walk.

Right now, I encourage you to pause with me. Ask yourself whether you can make a commitment *to yourself* to set aside time to not merely read it, but to reflect on it, alone and with those you care about. Make the time to do the practices that can allow you to begin to experience, within your own body and life, what it means to live the life you were born to live.

And from this very place, let's turn the page together.

Here and now, with faith, let's begin again.

—Rhonda V. Magee
January 2024
San Francisco, California

Introduction

This book is an offering for every person who finds an attraction to its pages and title. If you're curious about how to enhance your health, well-being, and capacity for joy by enhancing how you cope with stress, then this book is for you. It has been a labor of love to engage deeply in writing this book. The themes are partially reflective of my own personal journey, as well as the journeys of the many women who have shaped my life, including family, mentors, friends, mentees, and those I observed over the years from up close and from afar.

The most important thing I want you to know is that I believe you can experience a life of joy and wellness. In fact, I'm confident that you can. You can achieve success on your journey to health…including mind, body, and spiritual health. You can have healthy relationships, you can have career satisfaction, and you can have deep, soul-stirring, nurturing relationships. The first relationship for you to nurture is the one you have with yourself.

We are all on a journey of self-discovery, self-care, and *self-actualization*—self-actualization means to be the best possible version of ourselves. However, your success may be tied closely to the success of those you love—your family members, friends, and loved ones. Quite possibly, you dedicate yourself to ensuring their well-being so much that you leave yourself off your own to-do list. You might even continue to neglect yourself until you receive an alarming wake-up call that may include physical, emotional, or interpersonal suffering or pain.

You may see the signs all around you. There may be women in your life who gave all of their energy for the betterment of others. They ignored silent—and then not-so-silent—symptoms that they, too, needed attention and nurturing. But perhaps these women were too busy caregiving, and they forgot to care for themselves. Perhaps they were caring for so many others and didn't know how to care without carrying the load of those they loved. In fact, you may notice that you have a lot in common with these women. Yet how do you disentangle others' needs from your own? How can you care without carrying everyone else's "stuff" everywhere you go? How do you make your load lighter and easier to bear without neglecting those you love and care for?

You may even wonder, *When is it okay to take time to think about my own well-being?* It *is* permissible to prioritize your own health. It's *not* selfish to focus on self-care. As caregivers and supporters of others, making time to understand how to sustain your own health is actually an act of generosity. You cannot optimally help others if you're not well. If you cannot prioritize yourself for the sake of your own well-being, can you do it for those who are depending on your assistance? Can you do it for the young ones who are observing, taking in, and modeling their lives after what they see you do?

I was inspired to write this book because I've always been passionate about finding ways to help people be as healthy as possible. Quite frankly, I've always been curious about how stress can cause us to not be as healthy as we would like to be. While stress can sometimes be good, stress is often not so good. Stress can make us worried. Stress can make us sick. I learned this firsthand as a teenager and young adult.

Part of this is due to my makeup. I cannot ever remember not being a "can do" person. I always loved to help others. It's my natural inclination to raise my hand to take on a task, project, or challenge. This way of being brought on its share of stressors for me starting at a very young age. I've always possessed upbeat, positive, optimistic energy. I see the best in others, and I want everyone to win. As a result, I often found myself obligated to various organizations, committees, and other activities. This mindset also fueled my ambition to choose a career as a healthcare professional and a health researcher.

I knew I wanted to pursue a profession that allowed me to help others. Specifically, I was drawn to the field of psychology. I also felt a strong attraction to topics related to public health—keeping individuals, families, and communities healthy by focusing on direct patient care and community health, as well as through policies and laws. I was intrigued by the concept we now refer to as *health disparities*—disproportionate rates of illness among particular groups of people. My interest in psychology and health led me to ask questions such as: Why do certain groups of people experience certain illnesses more than others? For example, why were conditions such as heart disease, stroke, obesity, maternal morbidity, and preterm labor higher among Black women? I specifically remember wondering about what factors in their lives led to these undesirable health outcomes. I had a particular attraction to people's emotional well-being. What about their emotional or psychological experiences affects their health? What about their relationship experiences with loved ones affects their health? What about their environment or social experiences affects their health? What about how they experience and cope with the *stress* in their lives affects their health?

Little did I know, there was a professional field that aligned perfectly with getting answers to my questions—social and health psychology (or the study of how social, biological, and psychological factors influence health and illness). I first pursued an undergraduate degree in psychology at North Carolina Central University. Immediately after graduating with my bachelor's degree, I was accepted into a PhD program in social and health psychology at the State University of New York at Stony Brook (Stony Brook University). My first research experience as a doctoral student was working with Dr. Marci Lobel's Stony Brook Pregnancy Project, which focused on the influence of prenatal maternal stress (stress during pregnancy) on undesirable birth outcomes, including low birthweight and preterm delivery. Dr. Lobel's research study was one of the first to show that people with high prenatal maternal stress were more than ten times more likely to deliver their babies early compared to people with low prenatal maternal stress (Lobel et al. 1992). I worked as a research assistant on Dr. Lobel's follow-up studies on prenatal maternal stress and maternal-child health outcomes. During my first year of graduate school, I interviewed pregnant women to learn more about how psychological stress, relationships, and social factors influenced their pregnancy outcomes. With this indescribably rich experience, I had a gut feeling that I needed to expand my approach to my career. After much exploration, deliberation, and advice-seeking from family members and mentors, I decided that I wanted to pursue a career in nursing. I wanted to be more directly involved with the care of people I hoped to serve.

To make a long story short, I completed my doctorate degree in social and health psychology, a nursing degree, and an additional graduate degree to become a psychiatric nurse practitioner. Along the way to completing these degrees, stress related to managing school, work, and other obligations caught up with me. I suffered from emotional strain and physical health conditions so severe that I strongly considered quitting school. Thankfully, I had encouragement from my loved ones to pursue therapy for the first time in my life. The benefits of seeking counseling were enormous, and quite honestly, they continue to pay off. It was in therapy that I had my first formal introduction to mindfulness meditation. I learned how to show myself compassion through mindful awareness, which includes spending time in stillness with myself, paying attention to my own needs without judgment and with loving-kindness. I learned the benefits of respecting my own personal mind-body connection through meditation practices. I also had the opportunity to deepen my own personal spiritual practices by understanding and nurturing my personal needs. The core of who I am didn't change. My faith in God became stronger in deeply personal and meaningful ways. All the while, I continued to be dedicated to attending to the needs of others as a psychologist and as a nurse. However, I learned how to care without carrying the burdens of others with me all the time. I learned how to care while also tuning in to my own personal needs for care. I gradually learned to let others help me by expressing myself emotionally and seeking out the resources I needed to achieve my goals. I learned to prioritize my own needs, understanding that they were just as important as the needs of those I wanted to help or serve. I learned these invaluable lessons by engaging in many of the practices that I'll share with you in this book. Most of all, I developed a foundation of coping with stress that involved the seven pillars of mindfulness. Those seven pillars involve

- reducing the ways in which I judge myself or others;

- cultivating an attitude of patience with myself and others;

- approaching experience with the humility of a beginner's mind by seeing the world with fresh eyes and keeping my heart open to possibilities without being dangerously naïve;

- trusting my intuition and having faith that I will be protected and safe by showing up fully as myself;

- resisting the pressure to excessively push to make things happen while also having confidence and being my best self;

- accepting myself for who I am and accepting situations for what they are without become jaded or negative; and

- letting go or allowing my thoughts and experiences to be what they are, without judgment.

I learned how to see humor and beauty in the challenges I faced. I accomplished this by using all of the pillars to make positive changes in the world and fighting for fairness, justice, and opportunities for others without becoming completely overwhelmed or burned out from various sources of stress related to my identity as a Black woman who was trying to be her best in society.

I've continued to dedicate the bulk of my career to improving the health and well-being of people, with a specific emphasis on addressing the unique needs of Black women. It's my hope that this book will be a tool for meeting this goal. Hopefully, the content will resonate with you and have some degree of influence on how you can be your best self in the face of the stress you may be experiencing in your life.

I sincerely wish you well as you move along on your journey. I wish you joy and health today and for all your future days in ways that benefit not only you but also your loved ones and all who are touched by your life.

~Peace~

CHAPTER 1

Stress, Coping, and the Superwoman Schema in Black Women

Links to Health and Well-Being

When you hear the word "stress," what comes to mind? Stress is a common enough word, but what does it *really* mean? For many people, stress can be both good and bad. Being a little stressed can provide you with just the right amount of motivation to perform at your optimal potential. Stress can give you the energy you need to prepare for difficult tasks. Stress can help you do well on a test, a speech, or a job interview. Stressors that may be considered positive can include planning for complex events like a wedding or a milestone birthday celebration, purchasing a new home, or getting adjusted to a new position or a promotion at work.

Stress can also be experienced in ways that are not so positive. You may experience stress negatively, especially in situations that seem uncontrollable, relentless, or overwhelming. Examples of potentially negative stressors may include dealing with an illness; caring for a sick family member or friend; experiencing a breakup or the death of a loved one; or having difficulty at work, coping with financial strain, or enduring relationship challenges.

Stress and Health in Black Women

Did you know that stress is one of the leading health problems facing Black women? Researchers have found that chronic, unresolved stress can contribute to health challenges. You may already be aware of ways that stress affects your well-being. Stress may cause you to have a hard time sleeping at night. Perhaps you lose your appetite when you feel stressed. You may be a person who eats more when you feel stressed. You may engage in what is known as *emotional eating*, selecting comfort foods such as sweets or carbs to provide relief. Stress can lead you to experience sadness, depression, or even anxiety. Stress also can interfere with your ability to have healthy relationships. It can even chip away at your ability to experience happiness.

For some, stress increases risk factors for undesirable health issues. This increase can occur through engaging in unhealthy behaviors or through automatic biological processes that your body undergoes in response to stress. Stress can cause your heart to beat faster, and it can increase your blood pressure. Our bodies are less likely to be protected against exposure to the common cold when we are stressed. Our wounds may heal more slowly when we are stressed, and we may experience more physical discomfort or pain. When stress isn't managed well, our bodies just don't work as well.

We're also more likely to have chronic stress-related conditions. Some of these conditions that occur more frequently in Black women include obesity, diabetes, lupus, and cardiovascular disease. These conditions are not necessarily caused by stress, but stress may make them worse. Additional stress-related conditions that are more common in Black women include uterine fibroids and adverse pregnancy and birth outcomes, such as low birthweight, preterm delivery, and maternal hypertension. While there are multiple factors that increase the risk for these conditions in Black women, stress is a common link between all of them. Have you or any of your family members and friends had any of these health conditions? What are your thoughts about the role of stress in causing these conditions or making them worse? Do we have to live life this way?

Previous scientific research has found that Black women are at higher risk for these conditions because of the various *sources* of stress they are exposed to. Gender-related stress, which all women may experience, includes experiences of sexism, discrimination, or mistreatment simply for being a woman. In addition, you may indirectly experience or take on the stress experienced directly by your loved ones, family members, and friends. This is known as *network stress*, and it's more common among women. Black women have also reported exposure to race-related stress or discrimination, which adds another layer of stress over and beyond gender-related stress. Many Black women report distress related to being exposed to racism or sexism directly or when helping their children or loved ones navigate through experiences at school, healthcare settings, or social environments. It's possible that you've experienced gender-related or race-related stress, or a combination of the two (*gendered racism*), in various settings, including at work, where you live, where you shop, at school, or in social situations.

How You Cope with Stress Matters

Negative stressful experiences are often caused by inadequate resources to cope with the stress you're experiencing. When you have *adequate* strategies to cope with the stressors in your life, it's less likely that you'll experience symptoms of emotional distress. When you have *inadequate* strategies to cope with those stressors, you may feel overwhelmed, weary, burned out, or hopeless.

Financial resources, as well as family members and friends you can rely on to provide support, can help soften the potential negative effects of stress. However, these factors are often not enough. Emotional resources, such as resilience, spirituality, optimism, hopefulness, and even grit and determination, can go a long way in helping you deal with stress. However, challenges may arise when stressors accumulate from various sources. Situations that may typically be manageable can become unmanageable when they occur simultaneously, or if you're faced with one stressor after another in a relatively short period of time. A perfect example of this is how many people experienced the COVID-19 pandemic.

● *Natasha's Story*

Natasha experienced the combination of having to work from home while caring for her school-aged children and aging mother during the COVID-19 pandemic. Over a period of one year, Natasha had anxiety about avoiding illness for herself and others. Grocery shopping was particularly a chore and included a new step—wiping down each grocery item when she brought it home. Natasha witnessed loved ones get sick and even die from the complications of COVID. She experienced financial strain from changes at her job. The pandemic changed how her services were needed, so her paycheck became smaller. Natasha also experienced secondary trauma due to violence and racism against members of the Black community, including the killing of George Floyd and Breonna Taylor.

Natasha felt like her resources to cope with stress were first vulnerable, then altogether exhausted. Her usual coping strategies, such as going to the gym, enjoying a nice meal at a restaurant with her friends, or attending church service became less accessible or no longer available to her. She looked for new ways to cope with stress, such as gardening, baking, and doing puzzles. Although her new hobbies helped defuse stress that may have seemed relentless, the accumulation of stressors also caused her to adopt additional coping strategies that were less desirable, such as smoking cigarettes, drinking alcohol more frequently, sleeping more during the day, and becoming less physically active.

The social isolation Natasha experienced as a result of the pandemic increased her feelings of sadness, loneliness, and depression. By the time the pandemic started to resolve, Natasha's stress had caused her to eat more and become more sedentary, which led to a thirty-pound weight gain. This stress-influenced weight gain resulted in Natasha's being diagnosed with hypertension and prediabetes, and she developed insomnia. She also experienced symptoms of anxiety and depression, including worrying about the future, difficulty feeling safe when driving, guilt about things that weren't her fault, and loss of interest in things that previously gave her joy.

Do any aspects of Natasha's story resonate with you or another Black woman in your life? Even in times less dramatic than the height of the COVID pandemic, stressors from multiple sources can accumulate and influence your behaviors or your body's ability to snap back physically. Perhaps you've experienced symptoms of burnout, or you've come to realize that something has got to change. Perhaps you're aware of the potential dangers of stress in your life, and you're open to finding out what can be done to get your life back so you can experience joy and your full potential as a human being. You know that many types of stress are unavoidable, but you have a sense that you can protect yourself and your health. You're seeking longevity, happiness, and health, and you want to understand more about how to respond to stress in ways that don't create even *more* stress.

The Superwoman Schema: A Link Between Stress, Coping, and Health

Now that you have begun to think about how you experience and cope with stress may be influencing your health and well-being, it's time to think a bit more about the nuances of these relationships. Let's begin by considering a few questions. Do you take on the stress of loved ones, family members, and friends as if it were your own? Have you noticed that you ignore your own emotions, even neglecting your deepest needs and desires, to take care of everyone else's problems and needs? Do you avoid allowing others to help you? Do you reject help sometimes, thinking the person offering it may take advantage of you somehow? Do you find yourself pushing through what seems to be an endless flow of life challenges and hurdles to be there for your family and community? Do you find that you're tired of feeling tired all the time? Maybe you feel hesitant or guilty about taking a break from stress? Do you feel any level of resistance related to getting help from friends, loved ones, or a therapist? When was the last time you treated yourself to a deep level of rest, relaxation, and rejuvenation?

As you read earlier in this chapter, for some Black women, stress is made more complex by experiences related to race and gender. This may be why Black women have higher rates of stress and stress-related problems compared to many other groups. One challenge to how Black women manage stress in their lives is related to a concept called the Superwoman Schema (Woods-Giscombé 2010). The Superwoman Schema is a framework that provides information about how many Black women experience and cope with stress, based on their history, societal expectations, and familial experiences. The more you understand the Superwoman Schema, the more you will be able to understand and cope with stress to heal (or even prevent) its effects on your mind, body, and spirit.

The Superwoman Schema has five key characteristics that will be described more comprehensively in future chapters. For now, we'll start with a brief overview. The first characteristic is a **perceived obligation to present an image of strength**. The following quote illustrates one Black woman's thoughts about being strong. Does this resonate with you?

> *"I guess being a strong Black woman is doing what you have to do, like handling your business, taking care of yourself, taking care of what you have to get taken care of without complaining about it."*

The second characteristic is a **perceived obligation to suppress emotions**. Perhaps the perspectives in the following quote feel familiar to you.

> *"I try to talk about it but a lot of times you feel like people get tired of hearing your problems, you know. And people don't want you around if every time you come around you've got a problem. So you just keep it to yourself."*

The third characteristic is **resistance to being vulnerable or getting help from others**. The following quote illustrates why some women may resist getting help from others. Have you ever felt the way this woman does?

> *"It's hard to accept the support because of the things that are attached to it. Somebody asked the question about being able to let other people help you. And it's not so much that I don't want the help, but I don't want to give you an opportunity to think that I can't do it."*

The fourth characteristic is **motivation to succeed despite limited resources**. As you read the quotes, think about how often you feel the same way.

"My family expects me to do more than I have time to do,"
or *"Others get on me all the time, about slowing down, and*
I haven't managed that. Because I feel like I can do everything."

The fifth characteristic is **prioritization of helping or caring for others while neglecting one's own needs**. The following quote illustrates this concept. Does this sound familiar?

"I wish I could learn to say no because just about everything,
all the organizations, my church, family, whatever, I find
myself being delegated. These activities add more and more
responsibilities to my life. And I guess I'm not saying no strongly
enough. I like being helpful, but I am constantly putting off
my own needs."

The Superwoman Schema characteristics may cause you to avoid seeking help, which could cause higher or sustained levels of distress. Chronic stress may therefore result in physiological responses or health behaviors that increase your risk for depression, anxiety, or other stress-related conditions.

The characteristics of the Superwoman Schema didn't just appear out of nowhere. Some of the reasons you may have absorbed the characteristics of the schema may include (1) a historical exposure to racial or gender stereotyping or oppression, (2) receiving lessons from foremothers such as aunts, grandmothers, sisters, and mothers, (3) having a past history of disappointment, mistreatment, or abuse, and (4) relying on spiritual values that may be misinterpreted to mean that seeking help from a professional counselor or therapist may be a sign of inadequate faith. You might also consider how you take on these Superwoman

Schema characteristics to advance your current situation, maintain personal dignity, live a life of purpose, and "give back" to others.

Perhaps you perceive the characteristics that make up the Superwoman Schema as a double-edged sword with potential benefits and liabilities. You may relate to potential benefits of the Superwoman Schema, such as (1) the ability to survive challenging circumstances, (2) the ability to support the well-being of the Black community, and (3) the ability to support your family members and loved ones. On the other hand, you may also identify with perceived liabilities of the schema identified by other Black women, including (1) strain in your relationships, (2) stress-related health behaviors, including postponement of self-care, emotional eating, or poor sleep, and (3) embodiment of stress, such as anxiety, depressive symptoms, and adverse health. If the characteristics of the Superwoman Schema sound familiar to you, they may be robbing your life of joy, fulfillment, or well-being. If this is the case, help is on the way.

Hope and Healing Are Right Around the Corner

You're on the right path by finding this book and engaging with it. The book includes tools, resources, and guidance to better understand stress, the Superwoman Schema, and how they influence your mental health and well-being. Spending time with this book can provide you with what you need to manage and heal the effects of stress and live the life of your dreams. You have in your hands a guide to uncovering nuances of stress that may be unique to Black women. This book also will provide tools and strategies for gently and compassionately creating the life you're looking for. You're invited to engage in self-reflection and self-care, one step at a time. As each chapter unfolds, you will have the opportunity to explore personal stories of other Black women. Through engaging with their journeys, you will have more information to create a path to wellness that is uniquely yours.

Are you ready to move forward? The future is in your hands.

~Peace~

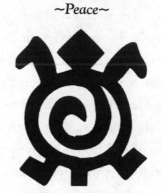

CHAPTER 2

Be Strong No Matter What

Are you someone who feels you need to be strong—no matter what? In other words, do you see it as *your* responsibility to be a source of strength for others, even when you don't feel like being strong? Perhaps you're constantly there for your children, your parents, or your partner. You may be known as the strong one among your family members or in your circle of friends. Perhaps you're the go-to person to solve problems at work; everyone depends on you to get things done. You feel that doing things right often requires you to be in charge. Being seen this way by others may feel like an honor at times, but it's possible that *always having to be strong no matter what may prove to be a source of fatigue or burden for you.*

In this chapter, I discuss the lifestyles of two women (Claudia and Monique) who represent the Superwoman Schema. Like many of you, Claudia and Monique experience a perceived obligation to present an image of strength for everyone. Their stories may help you understand more about being strong as one of the five characteristics of the Superwoman Schema—and what you can do to balance your need to be strong with your need to care for yourself. Each story helps illustrate how being strong may operate in your life and the circumstances that may influence your need to be strong. In addition, this chapter explores advantages and disadvantages of being a strong Black woman, because, as you know, this is both a strength and a quality that can wear you down if you don't bring awareness to it and find a way to harness its power in your life. With all of this knowledge, you will be able to consider the potential short- and long-term negative effects that this need to be strong may have on your health and well-being—and then learn how to maximize your strength without placing your health and well-being at risk. At the end of the chapter you'll find a meditation practice to help you begin to better *understand* and *optimize* strength as a personal characteristic that you can be proud of and that can support your growth and development as a person. With this key guidance, being strong can be a benefit (instead of a liability) for you. And, importantly, you will also begin to understand how to identify when it's okay to *let go* and allow yourself a break. It's okay to let go of that need to be strong.

● *Claudia's Story*

Claudia is a thirty-five-year-old mother of two daughters. Claudia considers celebrities such as Cicely Tyson and Oprah Winfrey examples of strong Black women. She thinks of strong Black women as regal, queenly, and determined. To Claudia, strong Black women "don't take any mess, and remain beautiful and dignified in all situations." So for Claudia, being a strong Black woman is definitely a good thing. It helps people around the world know that they can't trample on Black women or look down on them, despite stereotypes in the media of Black women as "welfare queens" or "poor, single Black women." Claudia feels that Black women have to be strong to let the world know all that they can do and be. Claudia also acknowledged that her inspiration to be strong came from her foremothers, including her grandmother. Claudia's grandmother was her hero. However, as Claudia reflected on her grandmother's strength, she began to wonder if being strong was also a source of strain and a risk factor for poor health.

"My granny had five children. She cooked and cleaned so that her home was always welcoming. Neighbors and church members often came by when my granny shared her large meals. She cared for her grandkids and volunteered at church, where she ushered, sang in the choir, and was on the community outreach committee. Granny was the matriarch of her family— when anyone had a problem, they went to her for assistance. She gave them help in any way she could, even if it meant doing less for herself. I never heard her complain. As I got older, I learned that my granny had high blood pressure, diabetes, and weakness in her legs and feet. Eventually, she had a stroke at the age of sixty, when I was eighteen. I never saw my granny cry (except for in church), but now that I think about it, her body did start to break down at an early age—from all those responsibilities. She was definitely a strong woman, but did parts of what made her strong also make her sick? I've always tried to emulate my grandmother, but now I wonder how I might need to do things a bit differently."

Unlike her granny, Claudia was able to go to college. She had her first daughter at age twenty and her second daughter at twenty-one, but she finished college nevertheless. She then worked two jobs while she attended graduate school. Claudia says this about her life now:

"There is just not enough time in the day to be a great mother, an excellent employee, and the healthiest woman I can be. I think I'm handling things wonderfully at times, and other times—most times—I just want to slow down and take a break. I wish I could make everything work, but I just don't know how. I'm afraid to consider that I might be turning into my granny in some ways. I get so much done, but at what cost? Will I end up paying for being a strong Black woman? I don't even know if it's possible to change. Being a strong Black woman can be good *because, you know, that's something you want to be called. Being a strong Black woman can also be a good thing because we don't let stress get us to the point where we give up on life. We just let it make us stronger, knowing that there's always going to be a brighter day, and that if it gets bad, then we can always give it to God and let Him handle it. I guess our faith is a lot stronger than other people's. I don't know why. And then it could be that...our stresses make us sick, make us have bad hearts and high blood pressure and all that stuff that comes along with our Black diseases or, not Black diseases, but what affects us more anyway. At least those are the diseases that affected my granny and took her away from us much too soon. Is that going to happen to me?"*

Claudia's reflections about her grandmother and about her own life may resonate with you. As a practice in self-care, it's important to stop and think about how we respond to life. Journaling is one way you can do this. As you read further in this book, you'll be encouraged to journal and reflect in various ways to get more insight about your experiences, which may help you cope with the stressors you experience and harness the strengths of the Superwoman Schema that are beneficial for you.

In a journal, reflect on these questions. Although the questions may seem to be a bit overwhelming at first, thinking about your responses will be an important step on your journey toward wellness, health, and joy.

- What are some qualities you associate with being a strong Black woman?

- Who in your life influenced you to take on the characteristics of a strong Black woman? Perhaps like Claudia, your grandmothers were a source of strength. Perhaps your mother, aunts, or other women provided examples for you on how to be a strong Black woman.

- Think about the women in your family and community who serve as sources of inspiration for you regarding how you raise your children, how you serve the community, and how you're there for others. Did your grandmother rise early in the morning and stay up late to get things done? Did you see her working in the home and in the church and displaying strength and resilience in every situation? Did she seem to remain strong, even in difficult circumstances? As those women displayed strength, did they also display engagement in self-care? What were the benefits of their strength? What were the costs of their strength?

- What about you? In what places do you feel obligated to present an image of strength? At home? At work? In your community? With your family? In your place of worship? In your organizations? In your circle of friends?

- What does strength look like when you display it? What are the benefits of your strength? What are the costs? Do you find yourself saying yes more than you'd like to?

- Most of the time, do you feel energized, or do you feel fatigued? Do you get seven to eight hours of sleep each night? Do you exercise at least thirty minutes a day? Do you eat healthy meals?

After you consider these questions, let's learn a bit about Monique. Her story can help us go a bit deeper in exploring this concept of strength no matter what.

● *Monique's Story*

Monique is a forty-nine-year-old Black woman. She has worked in her field for over twenty-five years and successfully moved up the ranks into management. As a result of her moderately high income, she has been able to create a nice life for herself. Nevertheless, Monique's work is incredibly stressful. She is the only Black woman in a management position. From her perspective, that means having to be perfect all the time—not only for herself but for the entire Black race! As she puts it, "I have to be strong; I cannot show any chink in my armor at work. Being a strong Black woman is doing what you have to do, like handling your business, taking care of yourself, taking care of what you have to get taken care of without really complaining about it."

Monique shared that being a strong Black woman is a double-edged sword. "My mother and father taught me to be strong. When I'm strong and people know that I'm a solid and reliable person, it's a source of pride. It makes me feel satisfied to know that I'm a key ingredient to the success and well-being of my coworkers and to the projects we develop and execute. I feel purposeful and more valuable, especially when people tell me how 'strong' I am. I wear it like a badge of honor. However, even though being strong may be a positive attribute, it makes me feel tired and stressed out to feel obligated to be strong all the time, especially when I face so many racial and social stressors. People don't expect to see someone who looks like me to be in the position I'm in, so I have to show up 200 percent. I feel like I have to be better than everyone else in everything I do. I must be on at all times. There is literally no downtime, and it's starting to wear on me. If I show any signs of weakness, I not only let myself down, I let my community down. Stereotypes about Blacks and

racism against us continue to be major challenges. I have to use
this opportunity; I have to show others that Black people are
more than they think we are. I can't let my hair down, like others
at my job. There is just no room for that. I have to be strong...
society makes me have to be a strong woman. Our past makes
us have to be strong women, and it's really annoying as hell."

The Need to Be Strong: Applying Claudia's and Monique's Stories to Your Life

Do Claudia's and Monique's descriptions of feeling obligated to present an image of strength resonate with you? You may feel a need to present an image of strength for the sake of your children, parents, siblings, or friends. You may find that, too often, you feel obligated to be strong in situations when you're feeling tired and out of energy. Nevertheless, you persevere.

You may feel that presenting an image of strength is just part of being a woman, and more specifically, just part of being a Black woman. The struggles of your ancestors may fuel your obligation to present an image of strength. Perhaps you feel like you need to be strong because of what your foremothers experienced during and after legalized slavery and systematic discrimination, such as overt and long-term racial discrimination, inequality, segregation, marginalization, and gender oppression, as well as social, political, and economic exclusion. Because of your ancestors' experiences with historical and societal stressors, you may perceive what they went through as much more challenging than what you're currently managing in your life. You may even consider that if your mothers, grandmothers, and other female role models went through struggles, you have no alternative but to be strong and go through struggles, too. You may consider this as your "lot in life," your "assignment," or your "cross to bear."

Being strong for you may feel like an asset or a survival mechanism for overcoming life's tremendous historical and continuing hardships. However, what may work well for you in the short run may eventually be a source of strain for you over time. While at first helpful, being strong may keep you from getting the support that you need and may cause you to have even higher levels of stress.

Religious teachings may also play a role in reinforcing the "strong Black woman" mindset and cause some people to take the role too far. Perhaps you've heard sayings such as, "God doesn't put on you more than you can bear," or "What doesn't kill you makes you stronger." These sayings are often shared to encourage people to get through tough times. However, as Claudia stated, "Although what doesn't kill you makes you stronger, what doesn't kill you can also make you sick." She was referring to a growing awareness about the strain that being "strong" can place on your body if it's not balanced with adequate time for rest and self-care. And that's what I want to turn to now. How can we balance this need to present an image of strength with our need to take care of ourselves? The key is self-awareness.

The Promise of Change Through Mind-Body Self-Care Practice

There are numerous mind-body practices that can help you recognize when these perceived obligations to present an image of strength are healthy, as well as times when they may be unhealthy. Strength can be *healthy* when it helps you get through challenging times or when it helps you achieve your goals. Strength can be *unhealthy* when it causes you to take on more than your body can bear. You may take on such a heavy load at work or at home that you incur negative physical symptoms. For example, you cannot rest; you don't make time for exercise; you've noticed your heart racing; your blood pressure has gotten out of control; or you've taken things so far that you've become physically ill and unable to do the things you want to do. Perhaps you don't realize that you've gone too far with being strong until you physically collapse with fatigue.

Yet, it's possible to be strong and healthy. By developing self-awareness—mind-body awareness—you can become more in tune with what your body needs and when it needs it. You can be wiser about when you can push yourself and when you need time for rest. With this awareness you can pace yourself. You can be strong without your strength becoming a liability. Your health can remain intact.

The practice of mindfulness can help you become more aware of any habitual patterns of responding to stressful situations you may have. For example, do you have a habit of staying up late and sacrificing sleep when you have major projects to accomplish? Perhaps you tell yourself that once you accomplish one project, you'll do better next time—and then you find yourself repeating the cycle of having a big task to do, then sacrificing sleep to get it done. You might even sacrifice healthy eating or exercising, only to find yourself gradually gaining weight, feeling moody, and regretting the process time after time.

With mindfulness practice, you also may be able to recognize when you're responding automatically with strength. Mindfulness practice can help you use strength in helpful ways, through recognizing the need for rest and reflection as you work to achieve your goals.

There are many different types of mindfulness practices that may resonate with you. Mindfulness helps you become aware of your thoughts and emotions. With it, you can learn what is driving you to take on obligations, and you can give yourself more space and time to decide what is most healthy for you. You can also learn to give yourself frequent mindful rest breaks when you're engaged in large projects, major tasks, or activities to achieve your goals. You can learn to embody strength that is sustainable over time—and in alignment with holistic well-being and fulfillment, rather than burnout and fatigue. Mindfulness can be in the form of rest breaks, as well as carried with you through all of your activities. When you conduct your life with mindfulness, rest, reflection, and resilience are integrated throughout your daily tasks, which can provide you with even more grace, poise, and a natural and energetic *flow* as you carry out your activities. This is how the Superwoman Schema and strength can become assets, not liabilities. Now let's try a practice called *sitting meditation* to help you build genuine, empowered strength that sustains, instead of drains, you.

Time for Practice: Sitting Meditation

Now is a perfect opportunity to practice what is referred to as *sitting meditation*. Sitting meditation is one mindfulness practice that can provide a restorative and imperative time-out for yourself to quiet the "shoulds" and "musts" that are often part of your need to be strong. Practicing sitting meditation may provide you with a sense of gentleness toward automatic reactions to challenges that constantly arise. The sitting meditation practice can help you choose to be strong in ways that are restorative. For example, you'll develop a sense of *body wisdom* that alerts you when it's time for a break from being a superwoman, or when you can allow your strength to flow gently with less pressure or wear and tear on your body. This practice is foundational to developing awareness of your thoughts and emotions. You learn to notice when you're judging yourself with messages such as *I should be doing this*, or *I should be doing that*; you can become skilled at releasing self-judgment. You can also begin to recognize when you're experiencing feelings such as shame and guilt about not being strong all the time. You can learn to recognize how these messages are causing you to push beyond your emotional or physical limits by having you say yes to things when you're probably overtired and overcommitted. You begin to accept that saying no or "not right now" may be a more appropriate response.

You can do the sitting meditation practice in almost any location at any time. All you need is your body, your mind, and your breath. Sitting meditation provides an opportunity to transition from busyness, which may involve focusing on numerous tasks and movement, such as thinking, planning, caring for others, and even worrying. This practice facilitates enhanced awareness of what's happening with you, in the present moment, *without* judgment. Sitting meditation is a practice that can help you cultivate genuine and empowered strength—the type of strength that helps you keep your head up, the type of strength befitting the queen that you are.

Step-by-Step Guidance for the Sitting Meditation Practice

Find a quiet place where you will be uninterrupted for twenty minutes.

Find a comfortable chair or cushion to sit on.

Sit in an upright posture or support your back while allowing your core to be a center of strength.

Drop your shoulders from your ears.

Hold your neck upright and elevate your head. Imagine there is a string attached to the crown of your head, and it's being slightly tugged on to uplift your posture in a way that feels dignified and composed, yet relaxed and without discomfort.

Close your eyes gently, or simply cast them downward so that you're not focusing on any one image or thing.

Allow your hips to be fully supported by the surface of the chair or cushion.

Notice if you're holding any tension in your hips or upper thighs and gently release any tension as you allow the weight of that area of your body to become lighter, as it's fully supported by your chair or cushion.

Perhaps even imagine that your hips or thighs are melting into your chair or cushion while allowing full support.

Continue to allow the chair or cushion to do what it is there to do, which is to support you.

Similarly, notice the surface your feet are resting on.

Gently notice if you're holding any tension at the bottom or top of your feet.

Allow the floor or surface to do what it's there to do—allow the weight of your feet to be supported.

Perhaps even imagine that your feet are melting into the floor while allowing full support.

Notice your hands and arms.

Allow your hands and arms to have a sense of support all the way down from your shoulders to the tips of your fingers.

Allow your hands to rest where they feel comfortable, perhaps in your lap or at your sides.

Let the weight of your hands be supported.

Bring into your awareness that at this time, there is nowhere you need to go, and nothing you need to do other than *be with* your body.

As you sit, notice what is going on with your body.

Allow awareness of your breathing to come into focus.

You don't have to change the quality or speed of your breath.

Simply notice how your chest rises and falls with each inhalation and exhalation.

Remain with the sensations of rising and falling in your chest area as you inhale and exhale for a few cycles of your breathing.

You may even notice the sensation of breathing in your upper arms. Gently expanding and contracting as each breath moves in and out.

It may be helpful to notice each inhalation and exhalation at the level of your belly.

You may notice how your belly shifts in and out as your body naturally takes in air.

You may notice the subtle movement of your lower back in coordination with the movement of your belly in and out.

That awareness may move up to your upper back.

You may notice the movement of the area around your shoulders and in your neck area.

You may even notice the sensation in your cheek area.

After a few moments of awareness in these areas, you may also notice your inhalation and exhalation through your nostrils, your neck area, and perhaps the gentle movement of your rib cage, inward and outward.

As you're sitting and breathing, you may notice your awareness shifting from your breath to your thoughts.

Perhaps you notice that you're thinking, planning, worrying, or even wondering when the meditation will be over.

Your mind may have shifted to imaginations or even a previous conversation.

If you notice that your mind has shifted to thinking, simply label your thoughts as "thinking" or "planning" or "imagining," without judging yourself or feeling bad that your mind has wandered.

Without attempting to control your thinking, simply notice you're thinking.

Then gently allow your mind to softly transition to awareness of your body's inhalations and exhalations.

Allow yourself to maintain awareness of the sensations of your body, with a friendly and easy approach, staying open to what comes, with curiosity and gentle, nonjudgmental presence.

Notice if you're starting to label your experience as pleasant...or unpleasant.

Notice, even, a tendency to judge your experience, and simply be with the experience as it is.

Perhaps you're beginning to feel restless or anxious.

You may be wondering when this practice will conclude.

Simply notice those thoughts or feelings arising, and allow your awareness to return to the sensations of breathing.

Notice how the sensations of breathing are different or similar in different areas of your body.

Notice the waves of breath...in and out...in and out...at your own pace and with a quality that feels most comfortable to you.

Notice if you have a desire to control your breathing to change the speed or the depth with which you breathe.

As you notice this, allow yourself to continue to ride the waves of your breathing as the breaths come and go.

If you begin to notice sounds, label them as sounds, perhaps noticing the quality, volume, closeness, sharpness, or length of the sound.

Gently allow your awareness of the sound to roll back to awareness of your breath.

You may begin to notice areas of your body that feel uneasy or uncomfortable.

You may notice the sensation of an itch on your body.

Allow yourself to notice the sensation and your body's response of wanting to scratch the area that feels itchy.

However, before automatically moving your body to address what may feel like an itch, allow your awareness to take in two or three cycles of breathing in...and breathing out...at your own pace and at your own rhythm.

After a few cycles of inhalation and exhalation, notice if the sensation of itching or the desire to scratch is still with you.

If it is, gently, mindfully, and slowly allow yourself to move your hand to the area of the itch to provide yourself with comfort.

Then gently allow your body to return to the original sitting position with your hands resting on your lap or at your sides.

As you're mindfully sitting upright, you may also notice tightness in your lower back or a desire to begin to slouch.

With mindful awareness, gently allow your body to shift to maintain an erect and dignified posture.

Perhaps allow your lower torso area to shift or move in small gentle circles or shift your pelvic area toward the front and then toward the back to allow your body gentle movement.

As you return your awareness to your breath and stillness, continue to notice the sensations of your chest, belly, and other areas of breathing sensation.

Notice your experience, without judgment, maintaining your attention on your breathing and simply being.

Reconnecting with the support of your chair or cushion for your hips and the support of the floor or surface for your feet.

Noticing your body as one breathing organism, present in this moment, fully and completely.

As this sitting meditation practice concludes, congratulate yourself for spending this time with you.

Notice your intentional awareness of your breath and your body and your curiosity about the experience.

As you sit for the final moments of this practice, honor this experience that is available to you at any time.

As you're ready to conclude, gently allow your body to start moving in the wise way that it knows how to do.

Perhaps begin to wriggle your fingers and your toes.

Perhaps lifting your shoulders up toward your ears, circling your shoulders backward and around, feeling the stretch in your back.

Perhaps allowing your head to slowly and gently shift downward with your chin to your chest, left ear to your left shoulder, head toward your back, right ear to right shoulder, and then again with your head toward your chest, before moving upright again.

Perhaps bring a gentle smile to your face, stretching in the ways that feel most comfortable for you as this meditation concludes.

Allow yourself the time and space you need to move into other activities of your day.

Time for Reflection

Now take a moment to reflect on all that you've learned so far from the words in this chapter and from your own personal meditation experience. Try to bring a gentle curiosity to how strength obligations developed for you and how they may be positive at times and less positive at other times. Use your journal to record the thoughts and feelings that arose for you.

→ In what ways does your strength mindset help you accomplish your goals? How does it also jeopardize your health?

→ What can you do to harness the power of your strength mindset—to have empowered strength that sustains you and allows you to accomplish the things you must do?

→ How can mindfulness practice be used to help you develop strength that is authentic, sustainable, healthy, and life affirming?

→ In what ways will you integrate sitting meditation practice into your life?

You can take the sitting meditation practice with you anywhere you go. It can be practiced at work or when you're in meetings. Sitting meditation can be practiced every day. Perhaps try it for a week, starting with just five minutes a day. You can even practice sitting meditation while you're waiting for your children to finish sports practice, or while you're in a waiting room for an appointment. Of course, you can also create a space in your home dedicated to your daily mindfulness practice. It could be a chair or cushion in the corner of a room, on your front or back porch, or anywhere that you feel safe and comfortable. Take some time now to plan ways to integrate mindfulness practice daily, particularly as you're working toward developing authentic, empowered, sustainable strength that fosters good health and well-being for you.

As you challenge yourself to practice every day for at least five minutes a day, write your experiences in a journal so you can see what comes up for you and how you grow during this process. At first it may feel weird to slow down and give yourself space for this practice. You may find every excuse in the book to not give yourself just five minutes for this practice. If you do, notice any resistance to practice and *do it anyway*. There is nothing to lose, and a lot to gain—for yourself, your health, and for the people you love. Just as you watched your granny or your mother, there are others who are watching you. Your journey to self-care is a gift not just to you but also to the ones you love. *Enjoy the journey!*

Conclusion

In this chapter, you learned about the Superwoman Schema characteristic, which refers to your need to be strong no matter what. You reflected on how this characteristic shows up in your own life, and considered who in your life possessed these qualities of strength. Maybe you saw yourself in either Claudia's or Monique's story, where you reflected on your own need to be strong no matter what and where this need comes up the most, such as in your relationships, in your community, or at work (or even images of Black women in media). For better or worse, you learned that being strong at all costs is an expectation that must be fulfilled generationally. No excuses.

While the Superwoman Schema in many of us may have been influenced by our foremothers, other factors may have been just as influential in determining for us when to project strength. Race, gender, racism, and sexism may influence your perceived obligation to be strong in many situations. These and other factors are totally out of your control, which is to say you need a tool that allows you to be strong in situations without jeopardizing your mental and physical health and relationships. This is where sitting meditation, as a foundational practice for developing new habits to prioritize being healthy in your life, may prove useful. With it, you're now ready to consider the other elements of the Superwoman Schema, and additional meditation practices that will support your journey toward balance, self-awareness, and well-being.

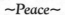

~Peace~

CHAPTER 3

Don't Show Emotion

Are you someone who feels you need to hide your emotions or keep them bottled up inside? Do you feel that it's best to keep your emotions to yourself? Perhaps you perceive crying as being a sign of weakness. Or maybe you have difficulty when you try to express your emotions. You may not show emotions in the ways that you experience them because you're trying to protect yourself. Perhaps you keep others from seeing your true self because you fear that they will ridicule or label you. Hiding your emotions protects you from getting hurt.

In this chapter, we learn about the experiences of two women (Pamela and Erica) who represent one of the five characteristics of the Superwoman Schema: a perceived obligation to suppress emotions. Like many of you, Pamela and Erica often feel that it's best to hide their emotions from others. Their stories help illustrate how suppressing emotions may operate in your life and the factors that may have influenced you to adopt this as a strategy of self-protection. In this chapter, you can begin to learn more about the strengths of emotional regulation without being in a place where emotional suppression causes you harm. It can be appropriate and in your best interest to hide your emotions in certain situations. However, constantly feeling like you don't have the freedom to express your emotions can result in emotional buildup and a situation where you may become overwhelmed or significantly emotionally distressed.

This chapter will provide you with tools for balancing your need to suppress emotions at times, while also learning ways to understand and work with your emotions. At the end of the chapter, you'll have the opportunity to engage with a mind-body practice, the *body scan*, to help you be in better touch with how emotions are stored in your body. Practicing the body scan can be a first step to avoiding undesirable effects of your suppressed emotions on your behaviors, your relationships, or your health. You'll also have an opportunity to think about the potential benefits of reaching out to a therapist or other trusted professional to start understanding the factors that cause you to suppress emotions, and how you may be able to resolve this challenge in a healthy way. Because emotional suppression is such a complex topic, you'll have other opportunities throughout this book to consider how other aspects of the Superwoman Schema influence this behavior, as well as additional mind-body practices that can help you feel equipped to manage your emotions in a healthy way. This chapter is only the beginning.

Let's begin this first step of the process to understanding emotional suppression by considering a time when you felt totally overcome with emotions or feelings of stress. Perhaps you experienced a need to cry, but you held back the tears and settled for having a major lump in your throat. Perhaps someone made you angry, but instead of expressing your feelings, you pushed them deep down into a place that only you know. What about those times when you felt disappointment or irritation? Instead of dealing directly with how you were feeling, you convinced yourself that it's better to hide what you were truly experiencing inside.

You generally may feel like it's best to suppress your emotions so other people don't see what's going on with you. Perhaps you hide your emotions because you want to protect others from also feeling stressed or upset. You don't want to be the Debbie Downer of your friend group, so instead, *you don't show emotion*. It's also possible that you suppress your emotions because you don't want anyone to think they have an upper hand over you. You may not trust others with your authentic feelings because they may respond in ways that are hurtful, invalidating, or even isolating. It's also possible that you don't want to be labeled as overly emotional, unstable, or even "crazy" for responding emotionally to situations. You may choose to hide your emotions because you fear they will be interpreted as anger or aggression (instead of sadness or frustration). Perhaps it's most important to you to avoid being labeled as an "angry Black woman."

Whatever your reasons, suppressing your emotions often comes at a cost. Have you ever been in a situation where your effort to hide your emotions backfired? You may have initially been successful with suppressing or channeling your emotions in particular situations but ended up exploding when you least expected it. Perhaps you keep yourself together at work or school but end up exploding emotionally at home with your children, partner, or other loved ones who are left bearing the brunt of emotions that were actually meant for someone else.

An alternative situation may involve loss of ability to express particular types of emotion. Lashing out or expressing anger may be how you release a broader range of emotions that are more difficult for you to process and unpack. There may be a series of situations in your past where you were unable to express feelings of disappointment, shame, fear, loneliness, or sadness. Perhaps you were concerned that people would interpret those types of emotions as weakness. This concern may even go back to your childhood. If you cried when kids picked on you on the school bus, you were at greater risk of being the victim of more bullying, so you learned to turn sadness into anger. When you felt disappointed by friends who were disloyal, you chose not to exhibit feelings of vulnerability. Instead, you felt safer demonstrating that you weren't bothered by betrayal or abandonment. You may have become aloof or tried to embody the trendy phrase "you're dead to me," even though losing the friendship actually made you feel grief, confusion, rejection, or loneliness.

It's possible that events in your youth generated emotions that were never processed. Like many, you may have been taught that children were to be seen and not heard. There may have been no safe place or clear mechanism for describing or sharing your emotions. It's possible that in your past, you were hurt by individuals, but it wasn't acceptable to communicate your feelings of hurt with them or about them. Perhaps a parent, teacher, or some other adult was a source of emotional distress, but expressing your true feelings was considered disrespectful or inappropriate. Perhaps you felt that you wouldn't be believed or validated, so you kept your feelings to yourself. You may have been told that anger wasn't ladylike, or that if you showed people your emotions, they would take advantage of you.

There are so many reasons why you may have developed a pattern of suppressing your full range of emotions. Let's face it, suppressing emotions can be totally appropriate in certain situations. If your supervisor at work says something to you that makes you upset, it may not be the best thing to "rip them a new one" by telling that person exactly what you think about them.

When your child has gotten on your last nerve at the playground, it may not be appropriate to yell at the top of your lungs to correct them. If you're completely frustrated with a waiter in a restaurant, name-calling is not going to make the situation better—it may even get you an additional, undesirable ingredient in your meal. When someone cuts you off when you're driving on the highway, flipping them off or rear-ending them may not be the ideal solution.

The actual problem with suppressing emotions is not that you don't—or feel like you shouldn't—*show* your emotions. The challenges come with *how* you channel or process your emotions. "Inappropriate" emotions may have been forced to be bottled up and packed away, but that doesn't mean they disappeared. For some reason you perceived your emotions as not permissible. Instead of being expressed, your emotions that were deemed unacceptable were stored in your body and in your subconsciousness. They weren't completely destroyed. Those emotions continue to exist because they weren't resolved. There may not have been space or time for you to process your emotions, even though they were valid for you to experience.

It's possible that you've become so good at suppressing your authentic feelings that you've lost touch with them. Now you're at a place of emotional numbness. This may involve cutting yourself off from situations or people who arouse unresolved emotions in you. You may avoid opening yourself up to emotional experiences that are difficult to manage. Instead, you may notice that you frequently experience bodily manifestations, including headaches; trouble sleeping; unexplainable chronic body pain, neck, and back tension; or an insatiable appetite for sweets and comfort food. Decades of suppressing your emotions may be an underlying cause of *avoidable* health problems, including (but not limited to) obesity, high blood pressure, depression, or anxiety. Let's take a look at Pamela to get a sense of the impact of not showing your emotions.

● *Pamela's Story*

Pamela is a twenty-eight-year-old woman who works in the nonprofit sector. Her work requires a lot of engagement with teams who are either internal or external to her company. She often must serve as a spokesperson for the community service activities that her company implements. Pamela's job involves a lot of stress, because of deadlines, reports, and consistent pressure to produce positive outcomes. Her coworkers depend on her coordination skills to achieve work-related goals. From the outside looking in, Pamela's friends admire the work that she does to help others in need. Pamela shared that no one seems to understand the pressures she experiences.

"When I'm most stressed, people often remark about how calm I look. But they don't realize that I actually feel like I'm crumbling inside. What they actually see is my game face. I feel

that I must hide how I'm truly feeling inside because, in the workplace, I'm supposed to be focused on being extremely productive. There is no time for displaying emotions. After work, I try to talk about how I'm feeling to my friends, but I'm scared that people will get tired of hearing about my problems. Also, no one takes my distress seriously because everyone thinks I have it all together, so I end up just keeping everything to myself. What I find myself doing is working long hours every day and releasing my emotions through food. When I get home after stuffing down my emotions all day, I eat comfort foods to resolve my stress. I love bread, sweets, and rich foods. Sadly, I often eat too much of these things. I feel guilty about it because I can tell that I'm gaining weight and that this is not the best way to manage my emotions. But food is just that constant source of relief for me—especially when I don't know what else to do to release the tension that has developed through the course of my day."

Time for Reflection

What elements of Pamela's story resonate with you? Pause here and respond to the following questions in your journal or notebook.

→ Have you ever been in a situation where you felt like people didn't take your emotions seriously?

→ Have you ever felt like you don't have time to express your emotions? When does this happen and under what circumstances?

→ Do you feel that others will feel frustrated, overwhelmed, or impatient with you if you try to share your emotions with them? What do you tend to do when this happens?

→ In situations when you hide your emotions, what do you do to find relief? Do you find yourself eating comfort food or overeating, like Pamela? What other behaviors do you engage in to release the emotions you don't share with others?

→ What long-term consequences of engaging in these behaviors could jeopardize your health and happiness?

→ What are you willing to try to produce a different outcome?

Let's take a look at Erica's story to gain more insight.

● *Erica's Story*

Like Pamela, Erica had become really good at suppressing her emotions. She hid her emotions from her coworkers, her family, and her friends for many years. Erica also experienced chronic headaches and insomnia. When Erica went to her healthcare provider to get relief from these symptoms, she also found out that she had high blood pressure. Her responses to a questionnaire she completed during her checkup suggested that she was highly stressed, which led her caregiver to suggest therapy.

Initially, Erica resisted the idea of going to see a therapist. She was concerned that if others found out, they would think she was "weak" or even "crazy." However, she felt that she had to at least try it out to find relief for what was causing her headaches, sleepless nights, and hypertension. Erica was getting to the place where she could not function with these symptoms. She had to do something about them. Fortunately, she was able to find a therapist rather quickly. Her therapist helped her understand that her years of allowing emotions to build up without releasing them had caused her current health problems. They also helped Erica understand why she felt a need to suppress her emotions. Erica realized that the way she had been raised was one factor that influenced her tendency to suppress emotions. The mother figures in her life were strong women who always hid their stress. Erica recalled several examples.

"My mom smoked a lot. It was her stress reliever. I didn't realize this when I was young, but I can see it now. We didn't have everything when I was growing up, but my mom made sure we had what we needed. Sometimes she worked two or three

jobs. She also went back to school so she could earn a better income and provide more for us. When I think of it, she was truly amazing, but she was always so busy. Despite all her stress, she never allowed us to see her upset. I never saw her cry. She even warned us not to let others see our stress, because they would take it as a sign of weakness. My mom hid her stress so well, but I did see her smoke... Unlike my mom, I don't smoke, but I have experienced holding in my feelings so much that I lash out at others who don't deserve it. I always say I'm sorry, but it's not fair for me to treat others like that. I knew that I needed to change to help relieve me of my headaches and sleepless nights and to keep myself from destroying relationships with the people I love."

Time for Reflection

Take a few minutes to reflect on Erica's story. What elements of her story resonate with you? You might grab your notebook or journal and spend some time responding to the following prompts:

→ What do you *know* about how you experience emotions?

→ How do you *label* your emotions when they arise for you?

→ Do you experience emotions that you feel are unacceptable? What do you *do* with those emotions?

→ What are the *underlying factors* that cause you to feel what you feel?

→ What kind of emotions do you tend to suppress? What type of *physical or psychological symptoms* may be related to the suppression of your emotions?

Change Through Mind-Body Practices

Like Erica, you may have hesitations about reaching out to a therapist or counselor to help you understand and process your emotions. However, it was only after reaching out to a therapist that Erica began to understand how her emotions were impacting her health and how her relationships had become strained as a result of her guarded behavior and emotional isolation. In addition, Erica's therapist taught her mind-body practices that helped her navigate her emotions and interrupt patterns where emotional distress led to unhealthy behaviors or adverse health symptoms. One practice Erica learned is called the *body scan*. The body scan practice was her first step toward understanding how she didn't actually separate herself from the emotions she tried to suppress. Erica shared that the body scan practice helped her see how and where she was storing her unshared emotions in her body. Eventually, she became comfortable with the practice and was able to release tension and emotions on her own. She became aware of when her unexpressed emotions were causing physical symptoms. After engaging in the practice on a regular basis, Erica experienced fewer headaches. She also was able to sleep better at night, and her blood pressure improved.

Perhaps, like Erica, you can also experience benefits from incorporating this practice into your life. The first step is to try it out. You may not experience benefits right away. You may question whether you're doing it correctly. You may even wonder if it's worthwhile. In this chapter, you have an opportunity to simply try it out. Try to minimize your expectations but do allow yourself to notice what happens for you.

Time for Practice: The Body Scan

The body scan practice builds on the sitting meditation practice that you learned in the previous chapter. As you try this new practice, remember that thoughts may come up for you. Gently notice what you're thinking and allow those thoughts to be released without judgment.

Step-by-Step Guidance for the Body Scan Practice

Before beginning the body scan, try to find a time and a location where you won't be disturbed for approximately thirty minutes.

Begin by sitting or lying down in a comfortable position.

Allow yourself to become aware of your pattern of breathing—not forcing your breath in any particular way.

Allow your eyes to take a break from taking in visual stimulation, perhaps allowing them to be downcast or completely closed.

Allow your hands to be at rest by your sides or on your lap.

Notice the rise and fall of your belly and chest with each inhalation and exhalation.

Then allow your awareness to go all the way down to your feet. Take in the awareness of each of the toes of your feet and their position on your body, noticing what's there. Remembering to breathe as you allow your awareness to move up from your toes to the tops of your feet, your heels, and the bottoms of your feet—encircling each foot and breathing as you notice any tension or discomfort there.

Moving up from your feet to encircle your ankles with awareness, gently appreciating this area of your body as you allow your awareness to move up to your lower legs, the fronts of your legs, and then circling around to the backs of your legs. Again, noticing what's there—any tension, any discomfort—and allowing your breath to encircle these areas of your body as you allow any tension to be released. Gently and gradually moving up through your knees and the upper parts of your legs, encircling your legs with awareness from the front to the back of your thighs and up through your hips and your lower back area.

Noticing if you're holding your breath and remembering to breathe as you spend a few moments with each part of your body. Allowing awareness and the flow of your breath to move up from your lower back, and from side to side through your middle back, up through your spine, and side to side through your upper back—noticing any tension or tightness in that area and releasing those sensations with each breath.

Moving up from your upper back to the lower part of your neck and across your shoulders—spending a little time to notice and release what is there, as you allow your awareness to move down from your shoulders to your upper arms, down through your elbow area, as you encircle and move your awareness down your lower arms to your wrists, breathing as you gently notice and release any tension there and move to the backs of your hands, with awareness moving through each finger, through the palms of your hands and back up through your arms and down your sides to notice your belly area, again sensing the rise and fall of each breath as your belly moves in and out.

As you notice what is there, remembering to breathe and allow your awareness to move up from your belly to your rib cage and chest area, perhaps taking in a deeper breath and releasing it as you move up through your sternum to your neck area and up through your chin. Remembering to breathe and release any tension with awareness as you move through your jaw area, encircling your ears, noticing your cheekbones, and encircling each of your eyes with awareness. Moving across each eyebrow, up through your forehead, and encircling your entire head with awareness from front to back and up through the top of your head. Allowing yourself to be fully aware of your entire body as one breathing being.

Conclude with gratitude for taking the time to spend a few moments with yourself. When you're ready, gently allow yourself to move slowly, perhaps by first stretching your fingers, pointing your toes, and allowing your eyes to take in visual stimulation once again in a way that feels most comfortable for you.

Time for Reflection

This may have been your first time experiencing the body scan practice, so consider the following questions in a way that is gentle and patient with yourself.

→ What did you notice as you engaged in the body scan meditation practice? (You may become sleepy or distracted when you first do this practice; these are normal initial reactions. When you do this practice next, gently return your awareness to your breath and the areas of focus on your body, as you allow any thoughts to be softly released.)

→ What did you notice about specific areas of your body? Did you sense any discomfort or tension? What else did you notice?

→ What experiences with your body allowed you to feel more familiar with it? What surprises, if any, did you have?

Conclusion

As it was mentioned at the beginning of this chapter, the process of understanding and working with your emotions is important, but it works best if you're gentle and patient with yourself. You may now understand a bit better why, when, and how you manage your emotions. Hopefully, you have more insight into the ways you suppress your emotions. Possibly, you have a bit more understanding about how suppressing your emotions may impact your mood, your relationships, and your body.

There is no need to have it all figured out by the time you finish this chapter. Your wisdom about yourself and your experiences will continue to unfold as you spend more time with this book. As you explore each component of the Superwoman Schema, you'll deepen your understanding regarding the factors that influence you to feel obligated to be strong and to suppress emotions. As you learn more a little each day, you'll open yourself to more opportunities to make gentle changes. The mind-body practices you've learned so far are available to you and can help you along this journey. As you continue to engage with the body scan practice, allow yourself the opportunity to discover new things about yourself and the ways you manage emotions. With each day, you will move along the pathway of self-understanding, self-acceptance, and wellness.

~Peace~

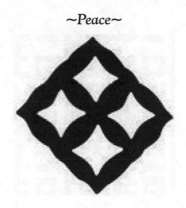

CHAPTER 4

Rely Only on Yourself

If you struggle with being vulnerable and depending on others, you're not alone. This may be one of the Superwoman Schema characteristics you can relate to, which means you probably have reservations about appearing vulnerable or feeling safe enough to let down your guard. At times, you may have allowed someone to help you with something and found yourself feeling disappointed or regretful for asking their help in the first place. Or maybe you asked for help, but then decided that to get something done right, you had to do it yourself. You may be concerned that if you ask for help, you will be unfairly judged or stigmatized as "weak" by others. Do you have a hard time trusting others? Or do you wait until you're overwhelmed to ask for help? Have you ever felt inclined to resist help from others to prove that you can achieve your goals on your own, without any assistance at all?

If any of your answers to these questions is yes, then you probably know what it's like to do it all by yourself and experience burnout related to stress. If identifying more strategies to cope with stress was one of the goals that attracted you to this book, it may be a good idea to use your time with this chapter as an opportunity for self-reflection. This chapter can help you set intentions and increase your awareness of how you may want to shift your thinking around asking others for help. Although it may feel daunting to even consider allowing yourself to be vulnerable or

"We don't want to let our guard down because we're scared to be hurt."

accept help from others, opening yourself to the possibilities of change this may bring in your life is a wonderful way to begin. You may be surprised that *there are people* who can be trusted, and *there are people* who take joy in helping you without expectation of anything in return. *There are people* who want to see you do and be your best, and *there are people* who will love you unconditionally, without any intention to harm you. *There are people* who have the intention to build you up and support your journey on this earth. Accepting these ideas as truth and visualizing receiving these gifts from others is an important first step to actually placing yourself in the position to accept support, encouragement, and love in your life. You're so deserving, so let's give it a try.

A resistance to being vulnerable and depending on others is a characteristic of the Superwoman Schema that can occur no matter what your age or educational background may be. In my research on issues relative to Black women, this resistance to help (and all of the other Superwoman Schema characteristics) were universal themes. Women shared the common experience of "putting up defenses" to protect themselves from being emotionally (and sometimes physically) harmed by others. Many shared that they didn't know how to accept help from others. There were many reasons for this resistance, including not wanting people to interpret their showing signs of vulnerability as indicators of personal weakness. It's important to recognize that being vulnerable and asking for help actually can be considered a strength! Others shared the importance of proving to others that they could make it on their own—without help.

Some women may resist being vulnerable and appear to possess supernatural strength and fortitude. Nevertheless, they may deeply wish they had someone to depend upon completely and consistently. But because they were hurt or disappointed when they gave someone the opportunity to help them in the past, they may be reluctant to be in that position again, and therefore continue doing what they have to do independently.

Black women who participated in my previous research studies reported reasons they resist help from others, and perhaps some of their reasons resonate with you. The legacy of stereotyping, racism, and sexism may cause some women to be suspicious of others and the help they offer. There is also the perception that people may assume that because you're Black and/or a woman, you're less smart or less able to do things that other people can easily do. Their offers to help may come off as patronizing, and any indication you may provide of needing help may reinforce their false stereotypes about your being inferior to others. In fact, their offers to help you may come under the guise of providing assistance, when they are actually threatened by the reality that you're not inferior but just as prepared and capable as anyone else, if not more so. Perhaps some of these experiences and perceptions resonate with you. Ask yourself, *Have I waited until I was overwhelmed or exhausted to ask for help and gone through challenges or struggles as a result?*

In this chapter, we'll use Angela's story to guide our discussion on the characteristic of shying away from asking for help. Like some of you, Angela resists asking for help or appearing vulnerable. I've included her partner Michael's story as well, because the two stories may help you understand more about how this Superwoman Schema characteristic operates in your life and how to address it. With their stories, we get to understand more about factors that influence the development of resistance to being vulnerable and receiving help from others, advantages or disadvantages of resisting vulnerability, and strategies to expand your ability to accept help from others.

● *Angela's Story*

Angela is a forty-five-year-old mother of one daughter. As a child, she witnessed the marital conflict and eventual divorce of her parents. Her father moved out of the home and eventually remarried. Although her father provided resources for her,

Angela spent the bulk of her childhood without a father figure in the household. She saw her mother make it on her own, and as Angela became a teenager, she and her mother survived challenging circumstances together through focus, hard work, and determination.

Teenage life with a single mother led to Angela's developing a relentless work ethic and sense of self. It also created a tough exterior for Angela that has lasted through adulthood. She is comfortable with controlling situations and being in a leadership role at work and in her personal life. Being in control provides Angela with a sense of security. From her perspective, being in control means not letting others help her and not allowing others to see any level of vulnerability in her. Angela believes that if she allows herself to be vulnerable to others they will be able to have control over her and over her life circumstances.

Unfortunately, some of her relationships only served to confirm her fears. Angela recalls when she fell in love with someone who seemed like her perfect match. Although she was certainly able to support herself independently, her love for this man allowed her to let her guard down. This boyfriend, who was quite financially secure, started helping her with her bills after they moved in together. However, that financial assistance became expensive emotionally. He started wanting to know her every move. If she took too long to come home from work, he questioned her about her whereabouts. If she bought a new dress for herself, he criticized her preferences in clothes. When she wanted to spend time with her friends, he reminded her of how much he was helping her and made it clear that her time should be spent with him.

When Angela started complaining about how their relationship was changing and suggested they go back to how *things were—Angela living on her own—her boyfriend told her she could not make it without him. He said that she needed him, and that her life would go downhill if she tried to live on her own again. Angela's independence became nonexistent, and her relationship with her friends was fractured. Despite the financial security the relationship provided, Angela realized that it wasn't worth losing herself. She ended the relationship and vowed never to allow herself to get in that type of position again. Still, the experience had lasting consequences for Angela.*

After years of going between being single and getting involved in short-lived relationships, Angela developed a deep friendship with a man named Michael. Like Angela, Michael had one child, a son, who lived with Michael's ex-wife. Although Angela was cautious at first, her friendship with Michael blossomed into a serious romantic relationship.

Michael occasionally brought up the prospect of marriage. However, Angela resisted any ideas about relinquishing the sense of independence that she had developed as a survival skill. She recognized that she had been taking care of herself since she was a teenager. Without the attention and affection of her father, she sought affection from her relationships, including an unhealthy connection to a boyfriend who had tried to control her. As a result, Angela once again vowed to never allow herself to be in relationships where she was vulnerable. She decided to take charge of her life, pay her own bills, and not accept help from others. Trusting others meant giving up control and being vulnerable, and she wasn't willing to make that sacrifice.

Although Angela understands why she tends to seek control in situations and avoid vulnerability, she sometimes regrets the way others see her. As a result of being self-sufficient, many people considered her aloof and cold-hearted. She was also called the term she disliked the most, an "angry black woman," because she avoided working in teams. For Angela, working in teams was a major source of potential vulnerability to others. She often did most of the work, while others took the credit. She wasn't angry, just self-reliant and protective of herself. Angela was afraid that if she shared her ideas, people would attempt to manipulate her or take advantage of her.

> *"It has hurt me to think people consider me as* angry *when all I'm trying to do is survive in this very unfair, and often oppressive, world.* I don't know who to trust in many situations, so I choose to trust myself. *I give others no room to attack me or get in the way of what I need in life. I remember learning the speech by Sojourner Truth in school called 'Ain't I a Woman,' and I identify with that so much. If no one is going to look out for me, then I have to look out for myself, and that's that. If I get called names or feel lonely sometimes, I'd rather choose that than to constantly get stabbed in the back by others who I thought would be there to protect or help me."*

Angela has a high level of self-awareness, yet it is clear that she also has a level of regret that taking care of herself also means being isolated at times and constantly on defense against being hurt by others. Nevertheless, Angela shared:

> *"But you know, I still want the people to want to support me. I don't want to give others the chance to think that I can't do something. If I were to open up to somebody, they may take my feelings and use them for their advantage. They may have ulterior motives for offering me their help. It's difficult to give up that control."*

As you can see, Angela is dealing with several complex emotions that are influenced by her past experiences with her father, her observations of how her mother coped, her previous experiences of letting down her guard and regretting it, and other situations where people tried to take advantage of her kindness, self-disclosure, or reliance on them. The accumulation of these events in Angela's life has made her feel that it isn't safe to allow herself to be vulnerable with others, so she has chosen to build a protective shell around herself. Inside, Angela wishes she could let her guard down. However, the fear of being hurt or mistreated is greater than her desire to have authentic relationships where she allows herself to be soft, delicate, and assisted. She resists opportunities to receive support from others, because she is uncertain about their motivations or what she will have to give up in exchange for support.

Angela lives constantly in survival mode, which causes her to miss out on experiences to partner with others at work or in romantic relationships. This self-protection that Angela exhibits is valid in some ways, based on her previous experiences. But like other characteristics of the Superwoman Schema, Angela's resistance to being vulnerable and accepting help from others is a double-edged sword. It also results in loneliness, resentfulness, and fatigue. This characteristic may also rob Angela of the opportunity to have a full relationship with Michael, someone who may actually be a wonderful partner for her. However, how can Angela know for sure that Michael's good intentions are pure? Should she take a chance? If things work out with Michael, Angela has a chance for a wonderful relationship. However, if Michael is like Angela's father or her previous relationships, she is at risk of being hurt and disappointed. Angela feels like she has experienced enough heartbreak, and she is not sure that she can afford to take the risk.

Resisting Vulnerability or Help from Others in Your Own Life

Perhaps you see yourself in Angela's story. Maybe you've been hurt too many times to allow yourself to depend on others. Perhaps you've decided that you cannot let your guard down and show vulnerability for fear that others will take advantage of you. However, you probably recognize that you need support from others, you just don't know who to trust or *how* to trust someone to help you. Is it possible to be protective of yourself *and* allow for vulnerability at times when you need support? Is it possible to be independent *and* receive help from others? If these scenarios are possible, how can they be achieved? Well, read on to see Michael's perspective. We'll find out how Angela's fear of vulnerability affected her relationship with Michael.

● *Michael's Story*

"I met Angela just a few years ago. I was attracted to her independence, her grace, and her ambition. Our energies matched, and from the first day I met her, I knew I wanted to get to know her better. I also knew that with a woman so independent and successful, I had to take my time to let her get to know me and show her that I had something to offer in a relationship. We enjoyed lunches, long walks, movies, and even quiet evenings at her house or mine. I really thought we were starting to build something that might lead to a long-term relationship, even marriage. I've been married before, and I knew that if I got involved with someone else, she would have to be special. This time, I wanted to have a relationship that would last.

"I noticed that when Angela and I would talk, even though we seemed to have a lot of chemistry, she would hold back from sharing her feelings with me. I sensed that she cared for me, but she never explicitly shared how she felt about me. I knew that she must be into me because she kept allowing me to take her out. We had good conversations about all kinds of things, like our careers, society, politics, and religion. We even discussed the goals we had for our individual children. We were both okay with the fact that her daughter and my son were our first priorities as we were raising them…things like that. I knew how I felt about her, and I even shared my feelings of love with her. One day, I even let go enough to tell her that I loved her. She smiled and seemed to really appreciate that. But for some reason, she was never able to share those feelings with me verbally. I started sensing that she was pulling back…pulling away from me.

"She always looked great, very well put together, but I also wanted her to know that she could relax and be free with me. Jeans, sweats, whatever… I wanted her to be able to be herself. But I never got that from Angela. After a while, it seemed like I was doing all the work of the relationship. I didn't know if it was fear or if she had just stopped caring for me. One day, I finally realized that this relationship wouldn't work, but before I could say anything about my feelings, Angela broke things off.

"My heart was broken. I just don't understand why I couldn't break through her shell. Her guard was always up. I tried so many times to help her see that she could trust me, and that I would never do anything to hurt her. I didn't say this, but I tried to show her. I still think about her to this day. She was a mystery…"

Time for Reflection

Reflect on these questions related to resisting vulnerability or accepting help from others, and write responses to them in your journal:

→ When you hear Michael's story after reading and thinking about Angela's story, what comes to mind regarding you and your previous experiences?

→ What experiences have you had in romantic relationships where it was difficult to trust and share your feelings?

→ In what ways did you miss a potential opportunity to develop and maintain a genuine and healthy relationship with a friend or with a romantic partner?

→ What about your past influenced these experiences in your life?

Perceived Benefits

Resisting help from others may seem beneficial for you, because it may provide a sense of protection from harm. For example, you may be concerned that when you allow others to help you, they will interpret their assistance as a license to make demands on you at a later time. They also may expect a level of closeness from you that you're not comfortable sharing. In addition, resisting help from others may seem to protect you from being characterized as vulnerable or weak, which could mean that others may see you as someone they can take advantage of. It's possible that you've been doing for yourself independently for such a long time that taking the lead or being in control of situations may be your default. Resisting vulnerability may give you a sense of control over when things are going to occur and what the outcomes will be.

This characteristic also is in direct opposition to stereotypes of Black women as being a burden to society. Through resisting help from others, you may be consciously (or unconsciously) attempting to demonstrate to others that you can make it on your own. You may be trying to show the world that you're gifted and talented, a contradiction to how many Black women report they are perceived—particularly in workplace settings. In addition, you may shy away from trusting others or revealing any signs of vulnerability because you perceive that coworkers, or even supervisors, will take any indication of vulnerability as a weakness or an opportunity to manipulate or discredit you. Keeping your guard up may shield you from misuse or abuse by others. This characteristic may be a source of survival and resilience for you.

Your perceptions are valid and commonly experienced by other Black women. Yet, there is a way to strike a balance between your desire to stay safe from harm and the ability to engage in authentic two-way relationships with others, while allowing opportunities to display vulnerability, receive help from others, and reduce the risk of emotional and physical burnout from doing everything on your own.

Challenges

Despite the many potential perceived benefits, resisting vulnerability or help from others can also have undesirable outcomes. This characteristic of the Superwoman Schema can cause isolation or loneliness in settings where support and camaraderie are critical for success.

Constantly being on guard to avoid being hurt or taken advantage of can be fatiguing and even confusing, especially when you're unsure who to trust in challenging situations or when you need a friend or mentor you can rely on.

Resisting vulnerability or help from others can impact the dynamics of healthy relationships. As a result of your attempts to protect or guard yourself, friends, family members, or partners may misinterpret your "tough" exterior as cold, icy, distant, uncaring, or inauthentic. As a result, people may mirror what they perceive as characteristic in you, and back away from revealing their own vulnerability, disclosing personal information, or asking for needed help.

Healthy relationships go both ways, with each person caring about and for the other. If a partner, loved one, or friend senses that they are not needed, it threatens the relationship.

> *"I think it comes with some bad. I feel like sometimes you have a tendency to be too independent…and you can turn people off from wanting to help you 'cause you're just so used to doing things on your own… We hold a lot in and try to fix it ourselves before we get help outside… We'll say, okay, I'll do it by myself. I can do this myself. I don't need your help."*

Although this approach may be used to provide protection from getting hurt, disappointed, or taken advantage of by others, it can also cause alienation from potential sources of needed support.

Resistance to being vulnerable or accepting help from others is associated with psychological and physical health symptoms and outcomes. Similar to other characteristics of the Superwoman Schema, the more likely a woman is to resist being vulnerable or accepting help from others, the more likely she is to report trouble sleeping, both in quality and quantity; lower levels of physical activity; more intense symptoms of stress and depression; and more frequent emotional eating to cope with stress (Woods-Giscombé, Allen, et al. 2019). So, if you resist being vulnerable and are overly self-reliant, you may need to examine how that impacts your everyday life and well-being. But first, let's look at how you may have developed this characteristic.

How This Superwoman Schema Characteristic Developed

Resistance to being vulnerable or accepting help from others may result from being in a previous abusive relationship. Angela's story is a helpful example of this:

"I raised my daughter on my own and refused to get into a marriage where I was going to be abused. During the last relationship I was in, I let myself be vulnerable with someone who mistreated me, so I decided that I was going to have my daughter and raise her on my own. I didn't want to give anyone else the chance to take advantage of me when I needed support, so I decided that I would not ask for help or depend on anyone else. Nevertheless, I would have loved to just have some 'me' time, you know, to not have to be the only one worrying about bills. My parents, of course, helped me; but having a partner who understood me and helped me so we could have made it without me and my daughter having to go through some of the things that we went through, that's what I miss. You know, you don't want to be strong all the time. You want to be able to be weak sometimes. But being weak and accepting help can mean being vulnerable with people who misuse your trust. It's hard to accept the support, because of the things that are attached to it... It's not so much that I don't want the help, but I don't want to give you an opportunity to think that I can't do it on my own."

And this can have a trickle-down effect. A mother who has gone through a struggle teaches her daughter how to handle that struggle without having to worry about it. And when her daughter has a daughter, she teaches her daughter. If this pattern is not recognized, it may continue through generations.

When reflecting on Angela's story, you may see that she was affected by many of these contributing factors, including experiencing her mom raising her on her own, emotional feelings of neglect when her father remarried and moved across the country, and feeling like if she wanted to be successful in life, she had to be self-sufficient and not give anyone any room to harm her. Michael, Angela's partner, didn't have the opportunity to know about Angela's history. As a result, he was confused about why Angela was emotionally distant. He took her approach to him personally, instead of understanding that she was trying to protect herself. This survival mechanism had both clear benefits and clear detriments for Angela.

Time for Reflection

At this time, it may be good to use your journal to respond to the following questions.

→ When you consider the factors that contribute to resisting vulnerability, such as feelings of neglect and the need to be self-sufficient, which ones resonate with you?

→ If you have ever resisted help from others, what may have been the cause for this in your life?

→ How did survival or self-protection contribute to your being guarded or emotionally distant with people who were trying to develop a relationship with you or show you love?

→ When you consider previous relationships, in what ways did you resist being vulnerable or receiving help?

→ What qualities does a person have to show you for you to feel like it is safe to show vulnerability?

→ When was the last time you allowed someone to help you?

→ If there are people that you allow to provide you with help, consider the reasons why you permitted them to do so.

Allowing the Gift of Support

Ironically, some Black women may feel obligated to take an approach to life that leads to isolation or loneliness, an approach that seems contradictory to the concept of collective support that Black communities have historically relied upon. Only a few decades ago, and still in some areas today, Black families and communities depended upon interconnectedness to survive the brutal environments of racism and oppression. Additionally, African cultural traditions that still influence the lives of Black people around the diaspora often include collective values. You deserve to experience the gift of support that you need as you pursue your dreams and goals, and all that your heart desires. Your journey to allowing healthy, authentic connections with others can begin with the *wise heartfulness meditation*, an expanded sitting and visualization meditation practice.

Time for Practice: Wise Heartfulness Meditation

This meditation involves the initial steps of sitting meditation that you learned in previous chapters, and then you're invited to envision the life that you wish to live. It can help you deal with fear. Resisting vulnerability and help from others is often grounded in a level of fear. Fear of being hurt, fear of being seen as weak, fear of being tricked, fear of being used or abused, fear of being manipulated, or fear of being disappointed or let down. Despite these, and perhaps other fears, your heart still longs to connect to others. As long as you resist the love and support that you deserve, you may feel isolated and perhaps incomplete.

Your heart can be trusted because your heart is wise. Your heart will attract authentic care from others if you allow it to be guided with wisdom. Your wisdom can be enhanced by allowing yourself to take a journey to understand the origins of your fears and to embrace what your mind, body, and spirit desire—true and authentic connection with others. By resisting vulnerability or help from others, you *may* be surviving, but at what cost? You may be robbing yourself of the joy, laughter, and deep satisfaction that can be achieved through determination to live intentionally with wise heartfulness.

The practice of wise heartfulness helps you protect yourself from potential harm without blocking healthy, authentic interactions with others. You can experience being grounded through meditation that allows connection with others in ways that won't threaten your safety. As the meditation concludes, you will be invited to journal what came up for you and what your clear intentions are for moving forward.

Step-by-Step Guidance for the Wise Heartfulness Practice

Prior to beginning the *wise heartfulness practice,* bring together the following items:

- A small table (or desk) with a tablecloth or covering in the color of your choice

- At least one photograph of your mother, grandmother, or the female relative who was most involved with raising you. (If you don't have a person who played such a role in your life, bring a photograph of the closest female mother figure, mentor, or loved one in your life.)

- At least one photograph of your father, grandfather, or the male relative who was most involved with raising you. (If you don't have a person who played such a role in your life, bring a photograph of the closest male father figure, mentor, or loved one in your life.)

- At least one live plant or flower in a pot, vase, or jar of water

- A stone, marble, or rock

- The earliest photo of yourself that you can find

- A cushion or chair

- A journal or piece of paper and writing utensil for the reflection component of this practice

Once you've gathered these items, you're ready to begin the practice.

Place the desk or table near a window or source of light in a quiet room or corner in your house.

Place the covering on the tabletop, then set out all the items listed above in an arrangement that feels best suited for you. Once you have the items arranged, follow your inner wisdom to add any additional items to the table. Listen to your inner guidance. It will tell you what to bring or to just use what you already have. Place your cushion or chair in close proximity to the table with the arranged items.

This setup is now your wise heartfulness space. This space can be set up as a permanent location for your meditation practices, or you can use items that can easily travel with you wherever it's comfortable for you to engage in this practice.

Make arrangements to be undisturbed for approximately thirty to forty-five minutes.

Take a seat, finding as much comfort as possible on your chair or cushion.

Lift your shoulders up toward your ears, circling your shoulders backward and around, feeling the stretch in your back.

Allow your head to slowly and gently shift downward, with your chin to your chest, left ear to your left shoulder, head toward your back, right ear to right shoulder, and then again with your head toward your chest, before moving upright again.

Allow the muscles of your face to relax, perhaps allowing a subtle, relaxed smile to appear.

Allow your upper body to move to an uplifted posture, allowing your core to be a center of strength.

Imagine that a string is attached to the crown of your head, and it's being slightly tugged on to lift your posture in a way that feels dignified, composed, yet relaxed and without discomfort.

Close your eyes gently, or simply cast them downward so you're not focusing on any one image or thing.

Allow your hips to be fully supported by the surface of the chair or cushion.

Notice if you're holding any tension in your hips or upper thighs and gently release any tension as you allow the weight of that area of your body to become lighter as it's fully supported by your chair or cushion.

Perhaps even imagine that your hips or thighs are melting into your chair or cushion while allowing full support.

Continue to allow the chair or cushion to do what it's there to do, which is support you.

Similarly, notice the surface on which your feet are resting.

Gently notice if you're holding any tension at the bottom or top of your feet.

Allow the floor or surface to do what it's there to do—allow the weight of your feet to be supported.

Perhaps even imagine that your feet are melting into the floor while allowing full support.

Notice your hands and arms.

Allow your hands and arms to have a sense of support, all the way down from your shoulders to the tips of your fingers.

Perhaps allow your hands to rest in your lap or at your sides.

Let the weight of your hands be supported.

Bring into your awareness that at this time, there is nowhere you need to go, and nothing you need to do other than *be with* your body.

As you sit, notice what is going on with your body.

Allow awareness of your breathing to come into focus.

You don't have to change the quality or speed of your breath.

Simply notice how your chest rises and falls with each inhalation and exhalation.

Remain with the sensations of rising and falling in your chest area as you inhale and exhale for a few cycles of your breathing.

You may even notice the sensation of breathing in your upper arms. Gently expanding and contracting as each breath moves in and out.

It may be helpful to notice each inhalation and exhalation at the level of your belly.

You may notice how your belly shifts in and out as your body naturally takes in air.

You may notice the subtle movement of your lower back in coordination with the movement of your belly in and out.

That awareness may move up to your upper back.

You may notice the movement of the area around your shoulders and in your neck area.

You may even notice the sensation in your cheek area.

After a few moments of awareness in these areas, you may also notice your inhalation and exhalation through your nostrils, your neck area, and perhaps the gentle movement of your rib cage, inward and outward.

As you're sitting and breathing, with your entire body, allow your eyes to take in the items on your table.

Scan across the table to take in each of the items while still sitting upright and breathing with your entire body. Notice any tension or any breath holding, and allow yourself to breathe with gentleness and grace.

Notice if any one item is attracting your attention more than others and spend time with that item or image first.

Allow yourself to pick up the item or image.

Notice what is coming up for you. What is the relevance of this item or image in your life?

Perhaps consider how old you were when you first encountered this item.

What thoughts are arising as you are present with this item?

What do you feel in your body as you are present with this item? Where do you feel it?

What lessons does reflecting on this item or image have to teach you?

Notice any particular resistance or openness that occurs as you are spending a few moments with the item.

Maintain a sense of openness and curiosity for what is coming up for you.

What emotions are present?

Notice if you're holding your breath to any degree.

Remember to breathe and relax any tension in your shoulders, jawline, or brow.

Stay with the item a bit longer and consider what being present with this item has to teach you.

Notice your heartspace—the area around the upper left side of your chest in the proximity of your actual heart. You may find that your heartspace expands across your chest and includes your entire torso area. You might even notice that your heart expands to your belly, your neck area, your face, your arms, your back, hips, thighs, legs, feet, and then all the way up through the top of your head and around your ears to the back of your neck.

In fact, you heart is interconnected with your entire body through vessels and tissues and breath.

Connect with your entire body and notice what messages may be coming up for you as you spend time with this particular image or item.

When you're ready, gently place the item back in its place on the table with a sense of gratitude.

Pause and allow a few cycles of inhalation and exhalation at your own pace and depth. Allow your fingers and feet to stretch, as well as any additional movement your wise body is encouraging you to do.

When you're ready, connect with the next item on the table that is attracting your attention, and repeat the previous steps.

One by one, engage in this series of steps with the subsequent items on the table.

Remain open to the experience. However, don't push yourself too fast or too far. Follow your own pace.

You will know when you've explored enough items for this meditation practice.

Once you've completed your engagement with the items for the current day's practice, remember to breathe and remember to smile.

Time for Reflection

In your journal or notepad, record what came up for you during the wise heartfulness meditation. You will begin to recognize how what came up for you relates to connectedness, vulnerability, and allowing yourself to receive help or care. Applaud yourself for engaging with this practice. Give yourself grace for what you achieved today, and when you're ready, return to the practice again to continue to engage with your items. *Enjoy the journey!*

Conclusion

Resisting vulnerability and help from others is a characteristic of the Superwoman Schema that carries a double-edged sword. On the one hand, it's a necessity with the purpose of providing self-protection, survival, and a way to not allow others to take advantage of you or harm you. In your case, you also may have come to recognize that you don't allow others to help you because when help is offered, it does not meet your expectations. We also discussed how resisting vulnerability and help from others may arise after previous hurtful experiences with people who offered help to you with strings attached. Or when you allowed yourself to be vulnerable, people perceived this as weakness.

Although resisting help and vulnerability may be a source of security and safety, you're also aware that not allowing others to help you can prevent you from experiencing authentic relationships or opportunities for collaborating in ways that may enrich your life either professionally or personally. Hopefully, Angela's and Michael's experiences provided insight that inspired you to reflect upon your personal life and the potential benefits of engaging in practices like wise heartfulness to understand factors that contribute to self-protection and to enhance your ability to connect with others in ways that are healthy and safe.

As you end this chapter, I also hope you now realize that you deserve an opportunity to fully experience your life in ways that allow you to be whole, strong, and vulnerable, yet protected and safe. The promise of this fullness can be fulfilled with enhanced self-awareness through the addition of wise heartfulness to the other practices offered to you in this book.

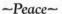

~Peace~

CHAPTER 5

Make a Way Out of No Way

Do you have a determination to succeed despite not always having adequate resources to do what you need to do? Perhaps you've made a commitment to "make a way out of no way." You may be someone who prioritizes being the best at everything you do—even when you're experiencing multiple stressors and barriers that could prevent you from accomplishing your goals. You may even put pressure on yourself to achieve certain things or high levels of accomplishments because others are depending on you to do so. Perhaps you continue to take on roles and responsibilities even when you're already feeling tired, stressed, or overwhelmed. If any of these circumstances remind you of yourself, then reading this chapter may help you understand more about yourself, while also providing you with an opportunity to consider how you can be your best without causing yourself harm.

"It's very important for me to be the best."

You may perceive numerous benefits to being able to make a way out of no way. You may have embraced this philosophy to survive difficult circumstances. You may see this as a symbol of your ambition and determination to overcome obstacles that could threaten your success. You may even feel a sense of pride related to achieving your goals. It's also possible that you get a sense of accomplishment from exceeding your personal expectations. You may be someone who has always had high personal standards. You want nothing less than the best for yourself, and this takes making the most of what you have in front of you.

"I work hard to prove others wrong. People have been ready to set limitations for me because I'm a woman or because I'm a Black woman. However, I know who I am, and I see so much more for myself."

Perhaps you feel motivated to exceed the expectations of others who doubted that you have what it takes to be as successful as you are in life. You may have experienced many situations throughout your life when people had preconceived notions about who you are and what you can accomplish. Perhaps you felt like you were placed in a box, and you decided to counteract the stereotypes and assumptions people have had about you. You committed to defying the odds or shocking others by showing them your worth when they underestimated your value.

As a result of your efforts, you may have achieved a lot in your life. Perhaps you're the first person in your family to finish high school or earn a college degree. You may be the first person in your family to attain certain professional or financial achievements. Perhaps you're the first woman or person of color to reach a particular position at work. You may be seen as a trailblazer. Because of your motivation and drive, exerting energy to overcome barriers and obstacles has been worth it to you and to those who look up to you.

"I'm used to being the best at everything I do. Doing less than that is difficult, and I literally get stressed out. I have no time for myself."

Despite the potential benefits of making a way out of no way to achieve your goals, this way of being also may be a source of distress for you. Your standards for yourself may be so high that you often feel frustrated that you're in some way inadequate. Perhaps you feel like you're not "enough" compared to the vision you have for your life. You may feel disappointed with *yourself* when it's your *circumstances* that have caused your limitations.

Being the first in your family to achieve accomplishments may mean that you didn't have parents, other family members, or friends to provide mentorship, resources, or guidance that others with more privileges may have had. As a result, your journey to success may have been filled with feelings of uncertainty, roadblocks, and hurdles that made things much harder for you.

You may even feel external pressures to succeed. Family members may be depending on you to "deliver" the family from generations of less-than-adequate circumstances such as poverty or undesirable environments. You may be expected to share your resources with family members or friends who have been less financially successful than you, and this may increase demands on you to continue to be successful despite unfavorable odds or challenges that are barriers for you.

It's also possible that succeeding in the face of limited resources increases demands on you related to your other multiple roles and obligations. You may have had to simultaneously juggle full-time work, complete your education, and care for children or parents with minimal or no assistance from others. This may leave you with absolutely no time to get extra rest or nourish yourself when you experience fatigue or signs of burnout. You may also not have enough time to spend with your loved ones or family members. While pursuing your goals, you may overlook that your relationships with family, friends, or romantic partners are being neglected or compromised.

So is it possible to achieve your goals for success while not completely overwhelming and exhausting yourself? Let's take a look at Camille's story.

● *Camille's Story*

Camille is a thirty-six-year-old mother of one daughter. Camille has always been ambitious. She was an honors student in high school and was awarded a full scholarship to college because of

*her academic achievements and extracurricular activities. She
came from a family of college graduates, but none of her family
members had gone to graduate school. Because Camille was
so verbal and analytical from an early age, her family always
declared that she was going to be a lawyer. Camille took on this
identity and made becoming a lawyer her goal.*

*Camille had the perfect life planned out for herself. She was
going to go to college, get into a good law school, become an
attorney, get married, have children, and successfully run her
own law firm. These plans changed drastically before Camille
completed her first year in college. During the first semester of
her freshman year, Camille continued to date her high school
sweetheart, who chose military service after high school. She
didn't yet know it, but Camille was already two months pregnant
when she started college. Although she felt disappointed with
herself when she found out about her situation, Camille became
determined that she could still achieve her goals. With the help
of her parents, she transferred to a college close to home. She lost
her full scholarship, but she took classes during the day and
worked at night so she could provide for her daughter. She
received financial assistance from her boyfriend, but it wasn't
enough, and she finished college with student loans. She was
admitted to a law school that had a program with evening and
weekend classes tailored to working adults. During law school,
Camille experienced several bouts of illness due to chronic fatigue
and exhaustion. Yet, with her parents' help, she was able to make
it through the challenging times and finish her law degree.*

*Camille was starting to build resilience. Overcoming the
challenges she encountered empowered her to believe she could
overcome future challenges. She figured that she could achieve
whatever she put her mind to—even if it meant that she would*

struggle or lose sleep. She was willing to sacrifice pleasures to reach her goals.

Camille became more and more determined. When she passed the bar exam, Camille received an offer to work for a law firm three hours from her home. It was the offer of a lifetime. However, choosing this position would take away the support she had been receiving from her family. Nevertheless, it would provide her with an opportunity to earn a great income to support her daughter and herself.

Camille was the first Black female hired in her department. Despite the potential challenges, Camille was aware that this position could be a great stepping-stone to future success for herself as well as for others coming behind her. Initially, she felt ready for the challenge. However, she didn't fully anticipate the challenges that were ahead of her.

Camille quickly found that her coworkers didn't see her as a peer, but instead as a person who was "given" a position because of her race. Camille realized that she had to work twice as hard at her job to be considered just as good as the other attorneys. She noticed that some of her coworkers seemed to benefit from mentorship or guidance from family members. Many were second- or third-generation attorneys, and here Camille was on her own. She didn't have trusted mentors or family members to give her tips for succeeding in this new world. She found herself having to leave her daughter at day care or with babysitters for longer hours so she could work into the night.

Camille was determined to show her team at work that they had not made a mistake by hiring her. She was motivated to defy the stereotypes they had about her. She felt like she was responsible for representing her race in everything she did in her position. Because so many of her coworkers had never *encountered other Black people with her educational level, Camille felt like it was riding on her to convince everyone of her worth. She also felt that her ability to make achievements in her position represented the capabilities of other Black people who might be recruited by her firm after her.* Camille felt significant pressure and stress. *Yet there was no turning back. She had to prove herself to the team against all odds.*

Fortunately, Camille's boyfriend's military commitment ended, and he was able to join Camille and their daughter in the new town. He was an excellent source of support at first— especially because he found a position with flexible work hours. However, when her boyfriend saw how much Camille was working, he encouraged her to slow down. He understood what was driving her, but his greatest concern was for their daughter's limited time with Camille and the burden that all of the stress was placing on Camille's health."

Time for Reflection

Perhaps use your journal to record your responses to the following questions:

→ What is your perspective on Camille's circumstances?

→ What parts of Camille's story can you relate to?

→ If you ever had to make a way out of no way, what do you remember about that situation?

→ Think about a time when you felt determined to succeed despite the potential consequences it would have for your health or important relationships. How did you handle the situation?

Waves of Stressors

Camille's ambition was fed by external as well as internal forces. When she was met with challenges, she found a way to stay focused and determined. The support she received from family facilitated her success. However, when she had less access to supportive resources and greater demands to be successful, Camille started to see the effects in more chronic ways. The writing was on the wall that if Camille didn't find a way to cope with increasing demands in the face of limited resources, she would continue to be challenged physically as well as emotionally. We have all seen this type of story so many times. Camille appears to be on the verge of sacrificing it all (including her romantic relationship) to achieve her professional goals.

Like Camille, we often see stress as a temporary struggle, with hope that once one stressor ends we will experience calmness and peace. Yet, if Camille opened her eyes, she would be able to see that she had been experiencing one stressor after another for a very long time. She was so determined to overcome challenges that this was becoming the priority of her life. She was so good at staying focused on defying the odds that she was losing sight of the other things in life that were sources of joy and fulfillment.

Life stressors are like the waves of the ocean. After one stressor comes in and goes out, another stressor is soon to follow. How we face stressors; how we cope; what we choose to sacrifice; what we consider nonnegotiable life values, practices, and traditions; and how we choose to navigate the process are all under our control. Camille had an option to not work at the law firm, which would allow her to avoid the stressors she was experiencing. However, being an attorney, a trailblazer, and an example to others was important to Camille. So, what did she need to do to achieve her goals? Is it possible for Camille to experience success in her current position while not compromising her family or her health? How could Camille begin to develop, access, and use resources that could help her have a less difficult journey?

How can you connect Camille's experiences to your own? Consider revisiting your answers to the self-reflection questions and identifying what steps you will take differently, based on what you know now.

● *Debbie's Story*

Debbie is a sixty-three-year-old heart attack survivor. At the age of fifty-seven, after many years of pushing through barriers and challenges in life, Debbie's determination and tenacity caught up with her. She had ignored warning signs of high blood pressure, fatigue, and weakness for many years until she had a major heart attack at work. After surviving bypass surgery to repair her circulation, Debbie went through a physical and emotional rehabilitation process that taught her a new way to live. Implementing new exercises and eating healthy became the regimen. She also began to work with a psychotherapist who helped her learn more about herself, including the identification of things that motivated her. She got insight into her emotional insecurities that led her to equate her self-worth with external accolades. Debbie was able to identify the things in life that were most important to her.

Debbie's heart attack didn't keep her from being ambitious. She learned how to listen to her body so that pursuing her purpose in life could be aligned with her personal well-being. She learned how to pace herself so she could make the most out of what her body could give. She learned to rest, and she learned how to seek out and use resources that were available to her.

Debbie's therapist introduced her to mind-body activities that facilitated this transformational process. Once Debbie became adept at using these strategies, she started a peer-support group to help other women like her—those who were ambitious but at risk for undesirable health outcomes because of their determination. She guided the women in her support group to engage in the practices she had learned so they could integrate them into their lives and avoid jeopardizing their well-being. She wanted to help them prevent major health events, like heart attacks, strokes, anxiety, or depression. When Debbie met a highly ambitious young attorney and mom named Camille, Debbie saw her younger self. Thankfully, Camille was open to learning the practices that had helped Debbie get back on the right track.

Deepening Your Mind-Body Connection

Perhaps like Debbie and Camille, you're open to learning to deepen your awareness and engagement with simple *mind-body practices* that have been shown by science to be effective for managing stress and preventing undesirable social, emotional, and physical stress-related outcomes.

In this section of the chapter, you will have the opportunity to learn about three practices: (1) breathing space, (2) mindful walking, and (3) mindful stretching. These mind-body practices can connect you to your inner wisdom and knowledge of how to experience wellness, even in the midst of ambition and stressors. With regular engagement in these practices, you may develop a broadened perspective about the mantra, or brief phrase, "make a way out of no way." You may be able to embrace the idea that these mind-body practices represent an array of resources available to help you live a purposeful life of fulfillment and actualization of your potential. As you're open to receiving these resources, you're invited to reflect upon how they can be tailored in ways that make them most helpful to you.

Step-by-Step Guidance for the Brief Breathing Space Practice

To familiarize yourself with the *breathing space practice*, identify a time when you don't feel rushed for three to five minutes and a location where you're unlikely to be disturbed or interrupted. Allow yourself to settle into stillness, feeling supported by your chair under your hips and the floor under your feet. Adopt an upright seated position that allows you to be as comfortable as possible. You may cast your eyes downward without focusing on anything in particular, or it may feel natural to allow your eyes to close. Allow what feels best for you.

When you're ready, allow your head to be in an uplifted position on your elongated neck with an open chest and expanded yet gently lowered shoulders. Notice your relaxed belly, supported hips, and the downward pull of your legs and feet, which are supported by the floor, ground, or a cushion. Allow your hands to rest without effort on your lap or at your side. Allow awareness of your natural breathing rhythm for a few moments, acknowledging that your body is supported and your being is safe. If it feels comfortable to you, inhale a breath through your nose and exhale the breath out through your mouth. In the moments of your inhalation and exhalation, consider bringing appreciation to this specific moment and acknowledge the time you're taking to engage in this breathing space practice.

If you'd like to try another cycle of intentional inhalation and exhalation, this time breathe in through your nose and allow a sound to be released when you exhale. It could be a loud breath sound or even a sigh. Do what feels best for you. If you have a history of respiratory illness (like asthma) or if some other factors cause this practice to be less comfortable, feel free to modify the process so that you can be present with a few cycles of intentional inhalations and exhalations.

If you find your mind starting to wander, acknowledge what your mind is doing and gently allow it to focus on your breath. Remember the principle of non-striving as you avoid forcing your body in any way, simply allowing awareness of each inward and outward breath as it feels comfortable for you to do so.

With each cycle of breath, perhaps bring a gentle smile to your face. At the conclusion of your practice, allow your hands to form a prayer position and rest them in front of your chest. Allow yourself to honor this moment and notice what you feel in your body, mind, and spirit. Feel free to accept the invitation to engage in this practice again to enhance your mind-body connection.

Step-by-Step Guidance
for the Brief Mindful Movement I:
Mindful Walking

To begin this mindful walking experience, allow yourself the comfort of supportive shoes if you're outside; if you're inside and it's comfortable and safe to do, you can do this practice with bare feet.

Prior to walking, allow yourself to stand in stillness. Noticing the connection of your feet to the ground, the energy in your legs holding up your body, the weight of your arms hanging at your sides, the upright curve of your back, the elongation of your neck, and the centeredness of your head.

As you prepare to take your first intentional step, lift your right foot to take a step and lower your right foot heel-to-toe to the ground. Notice the bends in your legs, the feeling of uplift in your leg, and the natural tendency to move forward by lifting your left foot. Noticing the bend of your left leg, the uplift assisted by your left hip, and the placement of your left foot to the ground heel-to-toe as your foot makes contact with the ground.

As you continue to take each intentional step, notice the motion of your arms, your advancement through space, the gentleness of the air on your face and across your body as you alternate picking up each leg and foot as you move forward through space.

Notice the contact of your body with your clothing and the swing of your hips with each step and rhythm of your gait. Notice the combination of lifting, swinging, lowering, as you move forward one step at a time. Notice your balance, and perhaps your feelings of being off balance at times when you move with such intention. Notice the twist of your spine and the concert of movements of various parts of your body supporting you as you walk. Perhaps even allow yourself to engage in a heel-to-head body scan, as you're aware of the placement of your feet, the movement of your legs, the swinging of your hips, the gentle motion of your pelvis, the gentle twists of your torso and spine, the upliftment of your chest, and the movements of your neck, chin, head, arms, and hands.

Notice the auditory stimulation; take in the sounds surrounding you as you engage in this mind-body walking practice. Notice your thoughts. Are you present with the movements, or are you thinking or planning? Notice your mood. Are you feeling any boredom, frustration, or gratitude? Acknowledging what is arising for you as your mind, body, and spirit are functioning. Continuing the intentional awareness of your walking for a few moments. And when you're ready for your walking to cease, gently finding a stopping place and allowing yourself to be present with your standing body in stillness. Noticing what you're thinking and feeling physically and experiencing emotionally. Allow the rhythm of your heart and breathing to settle as you gently acknowledge the time that you gave to experience this mind-body practice. As you form a prayer hand gesture and bring it to your chest, allow gratitude to flow through you as a result of the time that you spent showing yourself kindness and self-care.

Step-by-Step Guidance
for the Brief Mindful Movement II:
Mind-Body Stretching

Mind-body stretching practices can be as long or as short as you'd like them to be. The best thing to do is to start. Listen to your body for guidance on how to move. Your body will tell you what it needs. Remember to be gentle and practice non-striving.

It may be helpful to begin in a standing position with a gentle head roll. Allow the weight of your head to move in a circular motion, starting with chin to chest, left ear to left shoulder, head toward your back, right ear to right shoulder, and then again with chin to chest. Allowing at least four full rotations of your head in one direction, pausing with your head upright, and then circling in the opposite direction, chin to chest, right ear to right shoulder, head toward back, left ear to left shoulder, and chin to chest. After four full rotations, bring this movement to a gentle pause with your head upright, and move your awareness to your shoulders and upper arms.

Begin by allowing your shoulders to roll backward in a circular motion at least four or five times. Notice the release of tension in your body as you reverse this motion and allow your shoulders to roll forward in a circular motion. Then gently lift up your arms, allowing a larger circular motion moving in the forward direction, then reversing this larger circular motion toward the back. If it feels comfortable to you, gently lift your left arm over your head and stretch your body toward the right. Then gently move toward a standing position again and allow your right arm to lift over your head and curve toward the left. Lower your arm and allow your right ear to go more deeply toward your right shoulder stretching the left side of your neck, then gently switch sides and allow your left ear to deeply approach your left shoulder stretching the right side of your neck. As you are ready and able, move your neck back toward the center and gently allow your body to curve downward toward the floor, with your hands headed toward your knees or your feet, with a slight bend in your knees.

Allow yourself to rest here gently, feeling the stretch in your back and in the back of your legs, thighs, and hips. Noticing your breath, perhaps with awareness of tension leaving your body. Even allowing your upper body and arms to swing from left to right with the gentle weight of gravity. When it feels best to do so, gently allow your upper body to start lifting up to an upright position. Place your hands on your hips with your knees bent slightly, and gently rotate your upper body toward the right, to the middle, and toward the left. Returning to center and allowing the bends in your knees to straighten.

Create space between your feet as you clasp your hands in front of you, stretch your clasped hands forward, and then toward the sky over your head. Then gently allow your clasped hands to release, and guide them to slowly lower toward each side as you allow your chest to rise and fall with a cycle or two of inhalations and exhalations.

When you feel ready, position your hands into the prayer position and bring them toward your chest. Honoring the time you spent intentionally connecting your mind to your body. Gently feeling gratitude for this moment.

Time for Reflection

When you complete one of these mind-body practices, take some time to reflect and journal about the experience. Consider these questions:

→ What came up for you?

→ What insights do you have, if any?

→ What do you feel in your body?

→ What thoughts are coming to you?

→ How do you feel emotionally?

Conclusion

As you're beginning to familiarize yourself with these new mind-body practices, including breathing space, mind-body walking, and mind-body stretching, you may be wondering how engaging in these activities will help you attain your goals. What you may notice is that through these practices, you will gain insights into various circumstances and challenges in your life. Engaging in these practices on a regular basis will provide you with a gift of greater space for the many complex situations that you encounter. You may experience a heightened level of creativity and a higher energy level to address difficulties in your life. You may receive a greater level of clarity about what you need to make things run more smoothly for you. Engaging in the practices may help you be more organized or more open to new experiences. You may encounter aha moments that enable you to come up with solutions to otherwise challenging situations. You may have the wherewithal to identify a new mentoring team (regardless of your age or status in life), more efficient processes at work or at home, and a more joyous approach to each day. You may also develop a greater sense of self-awareness, which can help you prioritize what is most important in your life.

The gift of mind-body practices is an ever-unfolding opportunity for growth, insight, and wisdom. Where you previously saw limitations, you may now see new opportunities. With *regular* practice, you may have a deepened motivation to understand and achieve your goals with grace and ease. The practices are *always* available when you're open to engaging with them. They are your "way out of no way" and your boundless source of resources, self-knowledge, and inner wisdom. In aligning your mind, body, and spirit, you have an even greater opportunity to be the best possible you.

~*Peace*~

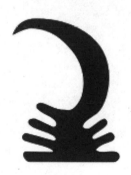

CHAPTER 6

Help Everyone Else First

In my research with Black women on stress and the Superwoman Schema, many disclosed feeling an obligation to be everything to everybody while putting themselves last. Many women also shared that they often take on extra roles and responsibilities when they are already feeling overwhelmed. They reported neglecting their own health and well-being to care for others, and they shared feeling obligated to say yes to requests. Granting these requests usually caused them to neglect their health or to neglect taking part in activities that bring personal joy. Black women who took part in my research studies shared feeling selfish or guilty when they made time to engage in self-care activities.

These feelings may resonate with you. You may have a need to nurture others, which is a common trait among women. You may even feel that it is your responsibility to make sure that everyone else's needs are met or that it is your job to make other people happy. Often being Black *and* being a woman creates challenges based on the social context of your life. For example, you may often be called to help others. This chapter includes examples of two women, Natalie and Sheila, who prioritized caregiving over self-care. Their stories will help you understand this Superwoman Schema characteristic, including

- why we do it;

- how culture prioritizes who gets served first;

- the benefits and liabilities of prioritizing caregiving over self-care; and

- strategies to use when you think there is nothing you can do.

Why Women Put Others First: The Experiences of Natalie and Sheila

You may very well feel that helping others is foundational to your identity, and certainly there is an undeniable degree of honor and appreciation we extend to others for their unselfish deeds and kindness. You may even think there is little cost for putting others' needs before your own. However, research on women helping others at the expense of nurturing themselves paints a different picture. There is nothing inconsequential about the consequences; they are literally life-threatening and necessitate a pause in the way we think about how we should care for others.

My research with Black women has revealed that putting others first is associated with psychological stress, insomnia, and depressive symptoms, as well as with emotional and binge-eating behaviors (Woods-Giscombe et al. 2019). What follow are stories from women who found themselves falling into a pattern of helping others while neglecting to show themselves the same considerations. We will see what happened to them in their efforts to keep peace in their homes, keep pace with life-defining moments, and make everyone else's life okay while they gave their own little attention. You may find that your own story is wrapped in theirs.

● *Natalie's Story*

Natalie is a Black computer scientist with a high-stakes career in security and defense. Her company initiated a workplace wellness campaign to help support the physical and emotional health of the team. This campaign was particularly important because of the high demands and frequent exposure to workplace stressors.

A mental health professional facilitated a company seminar on the topic of self-care, which frustrated Natalie. She later disclosed a major feeling of disconnection when the facilitator talked about the need to prioritize self-care over caregiving of other people. She shared that the facilitator seemed out of touch with the traditions of Black women. During an interview, Natalie stated, "I can take care of myself after I have helped the people I care about.

"Caring for them brings me joy and makes me feel good. It isn't possible for me to put my needs before theirs. That would actually make me feel bad."

However, as the seminar went on, Natalie reconsidered her perspective. For example, if she waited until all her loved ones' needs were met to tend to her own need for self-care, how could she ensure that she would be able to practice regular self-care activities, like healthy eating and physical activity? To understand Natalie's dilemma, we first have to understand Natalie.

Natalie came from a big family with three brothers and three sisters. Everyone looked to her for advice and support since she was considered the caregiver and the responsible one in the family. Natalie also had a daughter and a son, who were both adults but still fairly dependent on her for advice, and sometimes, financial support. In addition, Natalie's mother was becoming less physically independent and needed Natalie to take her to her biweekly medical appointments.

In time, pressure mounted for Natalie's attention outside the home. Her best friend, for instance, was in the midst of marital conflict and relied on nightly calls with Natalie for support and advice. So, although Natalie's idea that she would engage in self-care after she finished caring for others' needs may have sounded reasonable, in theory it was an impossible feat. There was never a time when one of Natalie's loved ones didn't seem to need her, and when Natalie finally had moments of quiet and time to herself, she found herself worrying about family members and friends.

Needless to say, the breadth of Natalie's caregiving robbed her of any potential peace and well-being. She eventually realized that to be adequately present for her family members and friends, she had no choice but to prioritize her own well-being. At first, prioritizing herself was quite difficult.

However, over time, she decided to integrate self-care with caregiving when she could. For instance, to get in more sister-time, Natalie would take walks with her closest sister; to ensure she didn't neglect her health, she shared in the healthy meals she prepared for her mother. With time, Natalie realized that it wasn't enough to integrate her self-care time with caregiving. She truly needed downtime where she could be quiet and reflective—and when she took this time, feelings of guilt and selfishness tortured her. Natalie thought to herself, Who am I to take time for myself when so many people need me? If I don't help others, then what do I have to give? This is the way I show love.

The workplace wellness campaign's next seminar was on the potential benefits of meditation for Black women. There, Natalie learned about how cultural values influenced by historical experiences with racism, oppression, barriers to financial resources, and resulting family-related challenges have caused many Black women to take on the role of caregiver for their families and communities. She learned that Black women are often perceived as the backbone of the Black family, serving as the glue that prevents complete fragmentation and destruction. Although being labeled as the backbone may appear to be a compliment, it brings undeniable costs to the emotional welfare of Black women, and it has sometimes caused relationship strain. Black women have developed an identity of the Superwoman who makes sure that everyone's needs are met, in the context of structural challenges that are of no fault of their own. For many women, thoughts about releasing any of this responsibility feel impossible. Nevertheless, Black women are deeply in need of the care they often freely give to others.

At the seminar, the facilitator introduced a potential key to ending the cycle of self-sacrifice: self-compassion, or treating oneself like a friend. Natalie learned that she could benefit from the concept of self-compassion. Through developing a loving-kindness or self-compassion meditation practice, she was eventually able to learn that being loving to others didn't mean having to sacrifice herself. However, given the many years of contrary information about her responsibility to prioritize caregiving over self-care, the lesson about self-compassion was a challenging one to learn.

● Sheila's Story

Sheila had gone months and months ignoring how tightly her shoes were fitting. She noticed that her ankles were often swollen, but she had no time to focus on that. Sheila had previously been diagnosed with hypertension, but she didn't recognize that keeping her scheduled appointments with her healthcare professional was a form of self-care. She often didn't notice her own symptoms of high blood pressure because she was focusing on everyone else.

For Sheila, the reward she received from volunteering in her organizations and supporting the happiness of her adult children outweighed any potential benefit of pausing to have regular health checkups. Eventually, chronic self-neglect caught up with Sheila. When she least expected it, she began experiencing severe tightness of the chest that would not go away. The discomfort became worse, and along with it, Sheila experienced severe fatigue and nausea. Understandably, these persistent symptoms disturbed her. She even thought about going to an urgent-care facility but decided against it because she simply didn't have time to be "waiting around in anyone's waiting room."

In her estimation, Sheila had "way too much to do." She was due to take her mother to an appointment, she was responsible for delivering donated clothes to the homeless shelter, and she was tasked by her brother to send documents related to their family's estate to the attorney's office before a certain date.

When Sheila arrived at the post office just before 5:00 p.m., after completing her other obligations, her chest pains were now at a level where they got her undivided attention. An attentive passerby noticed Sheila's distress and called 911. The ambulance rushed her to the nearest hospital, where the doctors told her she had had a myocardial infarction, commonly known as a heart attack.

Thankfully, after nearly one week in the hospital, Sheila was stable enough to go home. However, while she was in the hospital, visits with a social worker had also revealed longstanding mental health challenges, because she had no time to worry about herself when so many loved ones were depending on her.

Sheila's physician was aware of how much responsibility she had in her family, so she invited Sheila's children to participate in their mom's hospital discharge planning. Part of the planning *encouraged Sheila's children to give their mom time to recover at home. Three days after Sheila was discharged, her grandchildren's school was closed for a snow day. Unable to stay home from work, Sheila's daughter fell into old habits and asked her mother to take care of her three young children. Sheila, too, fell into her old habit of obliging her daughter's requests and agreed to sacrifice her own care to take care of three young, active grandchildren. Despite the guidance she had received from the physician, Sheila told herself,* It's my job to care for my family, no matter what. It makes me feel good to help.

Prioritizing Caregiving over Self-Care

Natalie and Sheila exhibited classic characteristics of the Superwoman Schema with specific, perceived obligations to prioritize caregiving over self-care. Historical patterns of racism, exclusion, and oppression have affected the educational, financial, occupational, psychological, and physical well-being of Black communities and families. Witnessing, and being affected by, these challenges may cause you to feel like you need to do more than your share to help your children, elders, or institutions that serve Black people. You may have a strong sense of responsibility related to "giving back" to your family or community. You may know that you *should* practice self-care. But doing what you know you should do may just not be part of your schema. This may keep your mind on serving others versus prioritizing your personal health and well-being.

Potential Challenges of Helping Everyone Else First

Although there are many benefits to caring for others, as Natalie and Sheila discovered, taking care of the needs of others may also cause *you* stress and damage your body. Your sense of commitment to others may make it difficult to say no when you actually have limited time or resources to share, causing you to take on multiple roles and responsibilities. And because you have developed a reputation for helping, new roles and responsibilities may get delegated to you. At times, there may be expectations (spoken or unspoken) for you to volunteer, whether you want to or not. Financial support of others may cause financial strain for you. Taking on multiple roles (or new responsibilities) may cause you to feel overwhelmed when you're already overcommitted.

One woman shared with me that "the problems of other people feel like excess baggage." What she experienced is a concept known as *network-stress*. Network-stress is related to stressors in the lives of family members, friends, or other loved ones. In contrast, self-stress is related to events you experience directly in your own life (Woods-Giscombé, Lobel, et al. 2016). For Black women, network-stress typically causes more emotional distress than their own stressors do. In other words, if your mother, father, brother, friend, child, or cousin is experiencing some life stress, you may be carrying their stress as if it were your own. The stress you feel may be related to worrying about or trying to solve the problems of those you love. This means that you may be experiencing way more stress than is reasonable for any one person to carry. Your load may feel heavy because of your care and concern for others. Is this healthy? Is this even reasonable?

Participants in my previous research study were aware that caring for others while neglecting self-care could have adverse emotional and mental health consequences. One woman shared:

> "I let myself have an [emotional] breakdown twice a year, and I do that in privacy. I probably need therapy; I surely could use it. But it's just then, I don't know how my life would be if I wasn't

putting out fires all the time. It just seems normal. That's just how it is. I just learned to deal with it." (Woods-Giscombé, Carthron, et al. 2016, 1137)

How Women Develop a Tendency to Help Everyone Else First

Many of the Superwoman Schema characteristics I mentioned before are learned from what you saw other women do. You may have witnessed your mothers, aunts, or other women in your community prioritize helping others while neglecting their own self-care. Women in my previous research studies shared numerous examples of how they developed a habit of prioritizing everyone else's needs over their own need for self-care. One woman identified the process as a trickle-down effect resulting from lessons learned in her Black community, where the role of caring for others was central for Black women. In her words:

> *"Big Momma went through a struggle, so she taught her daughter how to handle the struggle, so she wouldn't have to worry about it. And then her daughter has a daughter and teaches that daughter...and it continues."*

If you learned these characteristics because of watching others, who is learning them from you? Are your daughters, sisters, or sister-friends watching you and noting that caring for others means putting yourself last and jeopardizing your mental health and longevity? Is this the message that you intend to send? If your passion is helping others, will neglecting your own self-care eventually limit your ability to be of service? Will your legacy be unnecessarily limited?

Prioritizing Self-Care

Addressing chronic stress requires prioritizing self-care, and it's possible to *care* for others without *carrying* the emotional weight of others. As flight attendants instruct, it's important for you to put your own oxygen mask on before putting an oxygen mask on others. Caring for yourself is not selfish. Caring for yourself can actually give you the wherewithal to be of help to others in a more profound way. Are you ready to learn how to transform your reality to where you prioritize self-care *and* manage the ways you care for (and perhaps worry about) others?

Loving-kindness is a useful strategy for prioritizing needed self-care over excessive caregiving. The *loving-kindness meditation* practice can enhance your compassion for others, while also honoring your own need for self-compassion. It's a practice that can help generate feelings of caring and kindness for yourself and for others at the same time. In short, practicing loving-kindness can help you release burdens. Believe me when I say that it is possible for women to learn to "care without carrying" the burdens of others and the burdens of past stressful experiences. Through regular use of this practice, you can develop strategies to prioritize self-care, your own health, and your long-term well-being. In addition, loving-kindness can be used to promote mindfulness-based care for family, friends, strangers, and the entire world.

Loving-kindness is a practice that can help you learn to be gentler with yourself. This meditation can be used to cultivate positive emotions, including friendliness and compassion (Salzberg 1995). It can help reduce stress, guilt, and pressure related to caring for yourself as well as you care for others. Through this practice, feelings of being overwhelmed or distressed can be released. Loving-kindness meditation involves guidance that promotes connection with positive emotions. Purposeful attention is placed on directing loving acceptance and positive emotions toward specific types of people, including yourself; a respected, beloved person (such as a spiritual teacher); a dearly beloved person (such as a family member or friend); someone you know but don't have particularly special feelings for, like a cashier at the grocery store; a stranger; a hostile person (for example, someone you have or have had difficulty with); and finally, the entire universe. There are multiple approaches that can be used to boost feelings of loving-kindness, such as reflecting on a person's positive qualities and quietly reflecting upon brief phrases or mantras that can be utilized to cultivate positive emotions (Salzberg 1995).

Scientists have conducted rigorous research studies to investigate the healthful benefits and mechanisms of loving-kindness. They found that this practice is associated with reductions in chronic pain, emotional distress, and anger, as well as improvements in social connectedness, social support, and greater life satisfaction (Carson et al. 2005; Fredrickson et al. 2008; Hutcherson, Seppala, and Gross 2008).

Time for Practice: Loving-Kindness Meditation

For the purposes of this introduction to the loving-kindness practice, we will focus on self-compassion. The objective is to help you set intentions and priorities for engaging in daily work to promote health and well-being to enhance your overall quality of life. Later in this book, you will be provided with additional loving-kindness practices that can be focused on others.

Step-by-Step Guidance
for the Loving-Kindness Practice

Find a quiet place where you will be uninterrupted for twenty minutes.

Find a comfortable chair or cushion to sit on.

Sit in an upright posture or support your back while allowing your core to be a center of strength.

Drop your shoulders from your ears.

Hold your neck upright and elevate your head. Imagine there is a string attached to the crown of your head, and it's being slightly tugged on to uplift your posture in a way that feels dignified, composed, yet relaxed and without discomfort.

Close your eyes gently, or simply cast them downward so you're not focusing on any one image or thing.

Rest your hands gently on your lap or at your sides.

As thoughts arise during this practice, gently notice them, and allow them to be gently released—almost like releasing helium from a balloon. Don't push your thoughts away or resist them. Simply allow your thoughts to be, notice them, and then gently release them.

Now, notice your breath as it enters and exits your body.

You may connect with how your chest is rising and falling with each in-breath and out-breath.

Or you may notice the rise and fall of your belly as you inhale and exhale.

Breathe in a pattern that feels best for you. If you notice that you're holding your breath, perhaps three cycles of intentionally breathing in through your nose and out through your mouth will be helpful.

Then bring your awareness back to your chest or belly.

Notice your hips and upper thighs as they contact your chair or cushion.

Allow the chair or cushion to support your weight, then see if you can release the weight of your hips and thighs into your chair or cushion. If you notice any tension there, gently allow the tension to be released with each exhalation.

Similarly, notice your feet on the floor. Allow the floor to support the weight of your feet. You may even gently imagine the weight of your feet gently melting into the support of the floor.

Take notice of your body upright. Poised yet supported. Dignified yet comfortable, as your breath moves in and out.

Now bring to your awareness a person, pet, or group of individuals who consistently provide you with unconditional and unwavering love, kindness, and care. Allow the images of your supportive person, pet, or team to arise as if they were standing in front of you with smiles on their faces.

Receive the following caregiving message from those who bring you unconditional love:

_____(fill in your name in the blank),

May you be safe.

May you be healthy and well.

May you be happy.

May you be at peace.

May you always feel loved.

May joy constantly surround you.

Next, allow the images of your supportive person, pet, or team to arise as if they were standing slightly behind you on your right with smiles on their faces, and receive their caregiving message once more.

_____(fill in your name in the blank),

May you be safe.

May you be healthy and well.

May you be happy.

May you be at peace.

May you always feel loved.

May joy constantly surround you.

Finally, allow the images of your supportive person, pet, or team to arise as if they were standing slightly behind you on your left with smiles on their faces and receive their message.

_____(fill in your name in the blank),

May you be safe.

May you be healthy and well.

May you be happy.

May you be at peace.

May you always feel loved.

May joy constantly surround you.

Bring to your awareness a circle of loving-kindness energy that surrounds you as you allow your breath to enter and exit your body at your own pace.

Now, it's time to share messages of loving-kindness with yourself. Bring your hands to prayer position in front of your chest or cover your heart with your right hand and repeat the following three times:

> *May I be safe.*
>
> *May I be healthy and well.*
>
> *May I be happy.*
>
> *May I be at peace.*
>
> *May I always feel loved.*
>
> *May joy constantly surround me.*

At your own pace, continue to be aware of a few more cycles of in- and out-breaths.

Allow your hands to rest gently on your lap or at your sides.

Allow your fingers to start moving—perhaps roll your wrists around and around.

Curl and stretch your toes and feet.

Roll your shoulders forward, backward, and then up to meet your ears, down again, up again, then down to a relaxed position.

Roll your neck gently from left to right, from right to left, and then to center.

Gently allow your eyes to take in the scenery of the room.

Time for Reflection

Now that you've had an opportunity to engage in the loving-kindness practice, take time to reflect on your experience. What thoughts, feelings, or emotions came up for you? How do you feel after this meditation compared to how you felt before beginning the practice? Is this an activity that feels like it will be useful to you? In what ways might you incorporate it into your life on a regular basis?

As you further reflect, consider the first steps you can take to prioritize your own self-care. If putting others first has become habitual for you, what resources do you need to adjust this pattern so that it doesn't lead to premature burnout? Would it be helpful to identify a friend or buddy—another Black woman in your life, perhaps—to partner with in making changes in this area? Perhaps it would be beneficial for you to consider talking to a health coach or counselor to identify underlying factors that cause you to consider self-care as selfish or overindulgent rather than a necessary lifestyle habit for survival and resilience. If you find yourself constantly worrying about others, consider how this pattern of thinking may rob you of moments of joy, relaxation, or peace. The serenity prayer that is typically used to celebrate recovery offers the suggestion to "accept the things [you] cannot change" with a plea for "courage to change the things [you] can" and "the wisdom to know the difference."

Practicing all the mindfulness meditations introduced in this book may give you the space that is helpful to identify what you can change and what you need to let go of so that you have reserved energy to invest in your own healing and well-being. Taking the necessary steps toward self-care may perhaps be the only way to make sure that you're happy, healthy, whole, and around long enough to be a positive influence on the people and communities you care for the most. Once again, caring for yourself while also caring for others *is possible*.

● *Cheryl's Story*

*"As a child, I always had a big heart for other people. I was
(and still am) what I consider to be extremely sentimental.
I thought about and cared for others often. I was known for my
thoughtfulness and kindness—often referred to as* considerate.
*Although these were regarded as desirable traits, they often
disabled me emotionally. My mother noticed how much
I thought of others and took on their burdens emotionally during
my childhood. In addition to reminding me of prayer and other
faith-based practices to reduce my distress, she was open to
trying other methods that would possibly help me.*

*"When she came home from one of her work-related trips,
she gifted me with what were called worry dolls. She explained
that I was to share my worries with each of the dolls before
I went to bed. She also told me that the dolls could help me
when I was having trouble sleeping because I was worried. I was
grateful for my mother's sensitivity, impressed that she recognized
how disabling my 'thoughtfulness' for others could be for me.*

*"Although the worry dolls helped a bit, they didn't provide
me with the relief from worry that I needed. It wasn't until
I began to have physical symptoms as an adult, such as
unexplained abdominal and chest pains, that I realized I was
taking on too much responsibility for things I couldn't—and
shouldn't—control.*

*"I didn't find true relief until I learned about loving-kindness
meditation. One specific target for this practice was the worry*

over my grandmother. My sister and I were her only grandchildren. After my grandfather died, she lived alone in their home, in a town over two hours away from us. Although she was in a community surrounded by longstanding family members and friends, I felt worried about her whenever I got ready to go to bed at night. I had a hard time letting go of my fears about her being alone. I came up with what I thought for sure was a great solution to give me worry-free nights. Excitedly, I shared it with my parents. 'Let's buy a new house, big enough for Nana to come live with us!' But my grandmother refused the idea, telling us that she planned to stay put in her own house and in her own community.

"Only partially accepting her decision, I continued to worry about her. I tried to ease my concerns by calling her at night and making frequent trips to visit her on the weekends. When I began a loving-kindness meditation practice, I realized that perhaps I could release my worries about my grandmother using the concepts in the practice. At first, I thought I was being a 'good granddaughter' with my excessive concern and worry, until I fully accepted that my worrying about her wasn't doing anything to help her—or me.

*"As the practice directed, I gently sent her messages of loving-kindness—*May you be well, may you be healthy, may you be at peace, may you be calm and at ease—*each night as I went to bed. Then I internalized those same messages for myself during my nightly practice:* May I be well, may I be healthy, may I be at peace, may I be calm and at ease. *As I sent these messages, gentleness, warmth, and even happiness overcame me, and I sensed that I was somehow transmitting that energy to my grandmother. I soon found myself able to release my worries and easily fall asleep.*

"Integrating the loving-kindness practice with my Christian-based spiritual beliefs also worked for me personally. I recognized that God was always watching over and protecting my grandmother, and my worries (or lack thereof) didn't change that. Loving-kindness practice gave me the opportunity to reflect on the literal uselessness of my worries, and even the damage they brought to my emotional and physical well-being.

"Once I was able to use loving-kindness, I applied it to other situations where I was working too hard to provide what I thought was love and care for others. I was able to realize that instead of stressing myself, I could do what was actually useful and feasible. I realized and accepted that I wasn't created to be the 'be-all and end-all' of any one person. In truth, it would be a sad day if anybody totally depended on me, because if something happened to me, that person would suffer a terrible loss. I learned to do what I could and then 'let go and let God,' enabling the goodness of the Universe to provide what that person needed. I felt relieved…lighter and more effective, because when I was able to help, I wasn't overwhelmed or fatigued. I began giving from a 'full cup' with energy to spare to help those I loved, while also leaving time and energy to attend to my own needs.

"In addition to caring for family members and friends, I'm a healthcare provider who mentors many students and provides healthcare for disadvantaged populations. Because of the kind of person I am, I will likely never be able to ignore my desire to give back to my community and help people who look to my leadership. However, through loving-kindness, I've become more aware of my limits as a human being. I can show myself self-compassion and more easily accept what I can and cannot physically do for others without all the guilt. I use loving-kindness *meditation to extend wishes for well-being to others and to myself. It helps me accept that it's okay to answer requests with a no. Saying no to make sure I have time to care for myself is not an act of selfishness. I no longer feel guilty when I decide to carve out time for myself. I realize now that self-care is an act of philanthropy because it gives me the wherewithal to help others. Self-care sustains me so I can be around to do the work I'm passionate about. Self-care allows me to be a healthy, whole caregiver without unknowingly sending the message that self-sacrifice is noble."*

Conclusion

With loving-kindness and other mindfulness practices, the cultivation of self-compassion can be a major foundation for becoming more peaceful with prioritizing self-care to reduce symptoms of emotional distress, including worry, anxiety, or depression. This can become a rewarding life ritual—with benefits for self as well as for loved ones.

The characteristic of the Superwoman Schema that involves helping others no longer must involve neglecting your own needs. With loving-kindness for yourself, you can integrate self-compassion practices that allow you to be a friend to yourself without draining yourself of the energy you need to care for others.

~Peace~

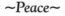

CHAPTER 7

Overcome Barriers with Self-Compassion

By now, you should be applauding yourself. You've made a serious commitment to improving your well-being and your ability to respond to stress in ways that can protect your physical and mental health. Now that you've been introduced to the components of the Superwoman Schema, as well as relevant mindfulness meditation practices, it's a good idea to understand more about how each practice resonates with *you.*

Are there practices that you enjoy more than others? When and where do you find it easy to practice mindfulness? When and where do you find it difficult? Are you finding ways to integrate these practices into your everyday activities? Perhaps you've started to notice barriers and facilitators to your personal ability to engage in mindfulness practices.

In this chapter, you will have an opportunity to identify those barriers that may create a sense of struggle for you. You will also become more familiar with the pillars or attitudes of mindfulness described in the introduction to this book, which can support you in deepening the relevance of mindfulness in your life. I'll share strategies for overcoming barriers to daily practice, including tips for finding simple ways to practice mindfulness in everything you do.

The overall goal of this chapter is to assist you with integrating mindfulness into your life in the way that suits you best. The best mindfulness practices are those you're able to do on a regular basis. You will also be encouraged to identify, prioritize, and schedule additional creative, reflective practices to generate mindfulness to enhance self-compassion and self-care. Lastly, you'll be invited to consider how you might expand your self-care toolkits with the mindfulness practices introduced in this chapter.

Although you've started to recognize that there are benefits of mindfulness meditation to enhance your emotional and physical health, you may still experience challenges to developing a regular habit of daily practice. There are common barriers that people face, whether they are new or more experienced meditators. Perhaps one of the following barriers resonates with you. If so, please know that you're not alone. Most importantly, please know that you can overcome it.

Five Common Barriers to Regular Mindfulness Practice

Barrier #1: The concepts of mindfulness and self-compassion still feel foreign to me.

Although the concepts of mindfulness and self-compassion may seem complicated, they are actually quite simple. Mindfulness is simply taking time to pay attention, on purpose, without judgment, and with heartfulness (Kabat-Zinn 2013). Self-compassion involves being kind and gentle with yourself no matter what. These ideas may seem complex, because you may have experienced an entire life of being told that you're most productive when you're busy. Perhaps you've received messages in your life that you don't deserve to be at peace. You feel more like yourself when things are challenging and maybe you've even learned to thrive in chaos. Self-compassion may be difficult for you because you may be used to being your own biggest critic or even your own worst enemy. You may be used to existing daily with thoughts of self-judgment, self-blame, or guilt. Perhaps you've always thought that you were never good enough and that you constantly have to be more and do more to be worth anything. Worse even, you may have been taught or influenced to dim your light. You know how special and gifted you are, but being your best self may seem to intimidate others or make them feel uncomfortable—so you tone yourself down so you won't stand out too much. You resist unwanted attention, but no matter what, you cannot avoid being seen for the beautiful and special person you are.

Whether you've come to believe that you're not good enough, or that you're too much for others to feel comfortable around you—you may be uncomfortable in your own skin. You haven't accepted yourself for who you are. These messages may have been passed down to you and internalized. Therefore, mindfulness and self-compassion practice may seem to be in conflict with how you previously learned to live your life. So not only are mindfulness and self-compassion foreign, but meditation practice may also be extremely *challenging* for you. These are the habits of mind that you're encouraged to simply *breathe through* during your formal and informal meditation practice. The practice of connecting with the breath is invaluable when thoughts of inadequacy, insecurity, or even uncertainty arise. Once you recognize a thought that may serve as a barrier to your practice, simply pausing with an intentional, slow inhalation and exhalation, followed by another slow inhalation and exhalation, may work wonders. As you breath in, try considering words that are affirming, such as "faith," "love," "joy," "enough"; even simply "present" may be helpful. When you exhale, allow any feelings of negativity, guilt, or self-judgment to be released. You may find that the more you breathe during your mindfulness and self-compassion practices, the less difficult these practices become. You may feel more natural with meditation and less connected to the thoughts or stories that are swirling around in your head, and more connected with yourself in the present moment. With mindful breathing, mindfulness becomes easier and more authentic and personalized for *you*.

Barrier #2: Focusing on the breath is a new and challenging concept.

Perhaps you've attempted to use the breath as an anchor to support your meditation practice, but you find that focusing on your breath is actually the part of the process that feels most difficult for you. You may feel short of breath, anxious, or even tense by trying to breathe *correctly* during meditation practice. Please know that this challenge is not uncommon. As children and even as adults, it's very likely that we didn't receive instruction on using our breath for health benefits. However, the breath is a core feature of our experiences of stress or anxiety. We tend to breathe in a more shallow way when we are tense or upset. We might even hold our breath or breathe irregularly, which can cause feelings of anxiety to increase—not just psychologically, but also physically. When our breathing is rapid, shallow, or irregular, it's likely that our pulse is also high, and our blood vessels might constrict. This will make us feel even more anxious. When people tell you to "calm down" or "breathe deeply," their good intentions may backfire and cause you to experience even greater tension. You might even have respiratory conditions, such as asthma, that may make it difficult to follow directions from others on how to breathe to generate calmness and mindful presence.

One useful strategy you can use to address the challenge of engaging in mindful breathing involves the development of an authentic mind-body connection. You can start by taking a seat or lying down and gently placing your hand over your heart or the center part of your chest. Don't try to do or feel anything in particular at first. Simply place your hand on your chest and notice the connection that is being made. Consciously allow yourself to be present with that experience, seeing if you can allow the other parts of your body to take a break or just melt into ease. You don't even have to change *how* you're breathing. Simply allow any strain or tension to melt away as you begin to notice the sensation of your chest rising and falling underneath your hand. With each rise and fall of your chest, you may begin to connect with your breath. But take your time. Don't force or rush the process. Allow yourself to just be with that experience for a few moments or even a full minute. Then, perhaps place your other hand on your belly—releasing the hand that is on your chest—noticing the rise and fall of your abdomen with each inhalation and exhalation. As before, you don't have to change how you're breathing at this time. Just notice, perhaps saying to yourself "breath in" and "breath out."

You may try this practice for a short time each day. It might be helpful for you to set a timer to support your breathing practice each day. Starting with a short amount of time may seem most manageable at first. Perhaps plan for two minutes, then three minutes, and then continue to increase the time by one minute each day. You don't have to be in a hurry to do more. You're building a new habit and allowing yourself to become more connected with one of the major components of your physical and emotional well-being—your breath. As you get more comfortable with this practice, you will be well on your way to maximizing the other aspects of mindfulness and self-compassion practice.

Barrier #3: The stillness of meditation is difficult for me.

Does sitting meditation make you feel restless, fidgety, or antsy? Do you feel frustrated with the stillness of meditation? You're not alone. Perhaps you feel like you're wasting your time. You have way too much to do and too little time. Sitting still is a luxury you cannot afford. You may even be uncertain whether you *deserve* to be sitting still. After all, there are so many people depending on you to be there for them. There is so much going on in the world that needs to be solved. There are people who need to be rescued. There is work that needs to get done. Your house needs to be cleaned. Bills need to be paid. Family and friends need to be called. Groceries need to be bought. A lightbulb needs to be changed. Your hair needs to be washed. Your lawn needs to be mowed. Dinner needs to be made. The refrigerator needs cleaning. The floor needs mopping. Birthday gifts need to be purchased. Thank-you notes need to be written. Towels need folding. Beds need changing. And on and on and on and on! How dare you even think that you have time to simply sit? As a matter of fact, sitting still is a waste of time. Or is it?

What if I told you that you could do all the things you need to do with more grace and more ease if you first take time for yourself with mindful meditation and self-compassion? Would you believe the research that suggests that practicing mindfulness helps make you feel like you have more time, more space, and more wherewithal to face the challenges of the day? Mindfulness practice can even make you feel more creative and allow you to approach your daily tasks with a greater sense of purpose and a heightened level of energy and ability.

But perhaps you were taught that "an idle mind is the devil's play-ground," and that the only way to get through life is to be busy and active.

Well, first things first. Mindfulness and idleness are not the same thing. Mindfulness and self-compassion are actually very active practices that can generate calmness or peacefulness; they are not passive practices that have no meaning or purpose. The practice of being present and nonjudgmental actually requires intention and focus. You're showing up for yourself!

The concept of automatic pilot can help you understand more about the active nature of mindfulness versus the passive nature of mindlessness. Automatic pilot is how you might allow your mind to operate without guidance or intention. If you pay attention to how your mind operates, you may notice that it jumps from thought to thought. Usually, these free-flowing thoughts are not very productive or helpful with regard to your wellness. You may notice that your mind has an automatic pattern (or automatic pilot) of visiting with a few habitual thoughts or even worries. You may be worrying about things that happened in the past, things you said, or things that were said or done to you. Or you may be worrying about what might be coming up in the future—anticipating things with worry, anxiety, or excitement. No matter if your thoughts about the past or the future are good or bad, you may find that you spend a lot of time in either place—the past or the future. Although this can have its benefits at times, being in the past or the future robs you of the gifts of the present—or what is going on with you in the present moment.

Perhaps take time to consider what is going on in this present moment. Well, for one, you're reading this book. Consider where you're sitting or lying. What room are you in? Are you outside? What are you wearing? What do you see, hear, smell, or feel? If you're eating or drinking as you read, how does your food or beverage taste?

Let's go a bit deeper with your experience of the present. Do you feel safe right now—at this very moment? Are you content? Are you taking in the fullness of what life has to offer? Think of the times you're present with your loved ones. When you're together with your parents, friends, children, or coworkers, do you take the time to totally absorb their presence and the connection you're making with them? Or do you allow the invaluable time to slip away by being distracted by the phone, the internet, the television, or other things that keep you from being fully present and receptive to the experience at hand?

The stillness that exists in mindfulness meditation gives you the ability to practice being in the present with what it has to offer. Granted, thoughts or feelings that you've been consciously or unconsciously suppressing may arise when you allow stillness. Could this be one reason that you've been resistant to slowing down? Are there things that you haven't allowed yourself to face because you're concerned about or afraid of what these things may mean for you? You may be resisting stillness and quietness because it's emotionally easier to crowd out things in your reality that are difficult to accept.

If this is the case for you, it may be helpful to welcome additional support for yourself. Despite the common stigma of allowing emotional support from others, this may be a good time to enlist a good friend, a clergyperson, or even a professional counselor to help you work through things you may have been suppressing for a very long time. These things just might be what has been weighing you down and keeping you from reaching new heights in your life. These may also be the things that are enhancing your experiences with stress and influencing feelings, such as anxiety or depression, or stress-related physical ailments. If you find that you're *avoiding* the stillness of mindfulness meditation, bring self-compassion to these feelings. Don't force yourself to do anything that brings distress, but do consider that this could be a sign that additional support may be just what you need. You do so much for others. It's perfectly okay to begin accepting help for yourself. After all, *you're worth it!*

Barrier #4: My mind wanders constantly.

A common concept in mindfulness meditation is *busy mind*. This concept actually goes along well with the concept of automatic pilot that you just read about. Courses in mindfulness meditation consistently remind those engaged to bring focus and awareness to the breath. This may leave you wondering, *What do I do with my thoughts?* You may believe that to focus on your breath, you need to quiet your mind by suppressing or avoiding your thoughts. You may even be telling your mind, *Stop thinking!* If you could somehow put barricades around your thoughts so that you could focus on your breath, this may seem like it would make practicing meditation much easier. However, this is exactly the opposite of what will support your practice. Trying to get your thoughts to stop is not the purpose of mindfulness. In fact, your mind is doing what it was actually made to do—*think*.

Thoughts are natural. The compassion you're attempting to bring to yourself can be targeted directly at your mind. Bringing gentleness and kindness to the thoughts your mind is experiencing can bring ease to the process of meditation. So instead of suppressing your thoughts, try *accepting* and *embracing* the natural activity of your mind. With gentleness, allow your awareness to connect with your body or your breath. Gently allow your thoughts to do what they do as they dissipate or move on from your central point of focus.

Time for Practice: Leaves on the Stream Meditation

One helpful practice that may resonate with you to become more comfortable with being gentle with your thoughts is called the *leaves on the stream* meditation. Let's try it.

Step-by-Step Guidance for the Leaves on the Stream Meditation

Take a few moments to find a space where you can sit or lie down comfortably without interruption for the next several minutes.

Once you're comfortable and supported by a chair, cushion, or some other surface, intentionally allow yourself to connect with your breath, by placing the palm of your hand on your belly.

Feel the rising and falling of your belly with each inhalation and exhalation—with each breath—perhaps using the words *breathing in* and *breathing out* to support this process.

Allow a scan of your body from toes to head and then from head to toes as you check in with your body.

Allow the weight of your body to be supported by the surface underneath you.

Notice sensations of tension or tightness melt away, and be supported as your breath circulates through your body.

As you become present in the moment and aware of your body as one breathing being, allow the image of a stream of water in nature to come into your focus.

You may begin bringing this image to your focus by noticing what is under your feet. Perhaps you're standing on a surface of earth covered by fallen leaves, pine needles, tiny tree branches, patches of grass, and dirt.

You're standing on the bank of the stream. Trees are shading the sunlight above you. You hear the chirping of birds who are both far and near. You notice the other side of the bank of the stream. And your ears and your eyes are taking in the sound and sight of the water flowing down the stream.

You notice how the water just moves down the stream. Nothing is pushing the water along. It simply flows, reflecting the light and the image of the trees as it moves along.

You notice objects moving downstream with the current. Pine needles and natural debris such as pinecones and leaves float along the water. You follow them with your eyes until they are no longer in view. You don't try to stop them or contain them. You just observe them as they move along the stream.

Some of these items flow effortlessly and rapidly down the stream. Other items flow down the stream at a slower pace.

You watch as some pine needles, pinecones, and leaves get stuck on rocks or tree roots that are impeding a smoother journey down the stream. They continue to move at their own pace, eventually becoming disentangled and flowing out of sight.

As you take in this scene, you may notice thoughts arising. These thoughts may be about the scene of the stream, or they may be completely unrelated.

You may be starting to become bored with watching the water. You may be wondering what is coming next. Or you may be unconsciously starting to make plans about what you have to do later in the day. You may even have thoughts of a conversation that you had earlier today and wonder if you said the wrong thing.

Whatever your thoughts may be, try not to judge yourself for your thinking. Try not to judge the thoughts, hold on to them, or push them away.

Simply take the opportunity to allow your thought to settle on one of the floating leaves, without trying to slow down the leaf or stop it. Simply allow your thought to be released gently, and observe its passage down the stream until it disappears from view.

You may fear that the stream is moving the leaves too fast to place your thoughts on them.

However, you can feel assured that you have all the time you need to place your thoughts on the leaves.

Some thoughts may float down the stream quickly and easily. Other thoughts will move more slowly, getting stuck in the debris or by rocks, tree roots, or other barriers—nevertheless, they will eventually float on down the stream.

You may wonder if it's okay to allow your thoughts to be released. Maybe you're having a good thought or an idea that you fear will be forgotten if you release it.

What if you never get that particular thought back?

Rest assured that this thought is part of you, and if it is worth holding on to, it will remain part of you until you're ready to bring more focus to it. You can choose when, where, and how you focus on your thoughts. Allow yourself to continue your time standing on the bank by the stream.

After some time, your awareness begins to lift higher and higher above the stream. You take in the scene of the stream, and then the branches on the shading trees, the tops of the trees, and then the sky above the trees, as if you were a bird flying higher and higher. As your awareness widens with the elements of nature, your thoughts are still present on the stream.

They just become less and less the center of your focus.

You become one living and breathing being.

Taking in the entire experience with your senses of sound, smell, feeling, and sight of the elements of nature around you.

Remembering to breathe, even remembering to bring a gentle smile to your face.

Eventually, you may find that it's easier to allow your thoughts to flow like the leaves on the stream—allowing your heart to be open to the presence of this moment, with awareness, without judgment. With full body awareness, heartfulness, and wholeness.

With time, strategies such as the leaves on the stream practice can help provide what you need to manage your thinking and engage as fully as possible in mindfulness practice. Remember to continue to practice patience and compassion with yourself—your thoughts don't have to be pushed away or stopped. With the acceptance of what our minds naturally do, you can allow your thoughts to flow like the leaves on the stream without being the central focus of your existence.

Barrier #5: I have a problem establishing a routine in the midst of my stressful life.

It's possible that the biggest barrier you experience to integrating mindfulness and self-compassion into your everyday existence is establishing a routine. Practicing mindfulness when you're constantly busy and on the go is indeed a challenge. You may have the best intentions to develop a habit of practice, but something gets in your way each and every day. With so many things on your plate and the occurrence of unexpected events, you may simply forget to practice. Thankfully there are solutions to this that are practical and achievable for you.

PUT MINDFULNESS ON YOUR SCHEDULE.

The first strategy is to set an appointment with yourself to practice. Just like you put everyone else on your schedule, make an appointment to engage in your mindfulness practice and place it on your calendar. You might even set a pleasant alarm that will alert you. It may be optimal to start your day with practice. That may keep you from forgetting. It can be like filling your car with gas before you can go anywhere. Your commitment to practicing mindfulness at the beginning of each day can be a powerful symbol of self-care for yourself, as well as for those who know and love you. Starting your day with mindfulness may also be a good routine to establish because you may feel too tired to practice mindfulness at the end of the day. You may find yourself falling asleep or avoiding the practice altogether, especially after you've had a stressful day. Of course, however, when you feel particularly stressed or uneasy, mindfulness practice may be the most useful.

INCORPORATE MINDFUL MOVEMENT AND THE BODY SCAN EVEN WHEN YOU FEEL TIRED OR STRESSED.

There are a few ways to integrate mindfulness and self-care practice into your day when you're feeling tired or distressed. First, you might choose to conclude the day with gentle mindful movement to help undo the tension that has collected in your body. A few mindful and intentional neck, shoulder, and arm rolls may help release the knots in your upper back. Gentle mindful stretching postures may help dissipate the stress that has built up in the other parts of your body and keep it from accumulating day after day. A brief walking meditation practice at the end of each day is also an approach that may help you de-stress and relax your body in preparation for an optimal night of sleep. The body scan meditation is a gentle way to practice mindfulness when your body is excessively tired. While breathing and focusing on sensations in your body from your toes up through your feet, ankles, legs, hips, back, neck, arms, belly, chest, neck, face, and head, you can give your body a mindful tune-up while enhancing your mind-body connection with little or no impact.

INTEGRATE MINDFULNESS IN YOUR CAREGIVING PRACTICES.

Some of the most common complaints about the challenges of integrating mindfulness practice into everyday life come from the sandwich generation—parents who are caring for their own aging parents or other loved ones. They may feel that they have absolutely no downtime to focus on their own health and well-being.

If you're a caregiver, the stress related to constantly pouring your energy into the health and well-being of others can be completely overwhelming and draining. You may feel like it's utterly impossible to get any time in for yourself. However, you have an opportunity to bring mindfulness to your caregiving activities. As long as you have your breath as a tool to assist you, you have the opportunity to practice mindfulness and self-compassion, as well as compassion for others. As a matter of fact, it's critical for you as a caregiver to become skilled at embracing mindfulness practice so you can survive this challenge of caregiving without becoming burned out or ill from the responsibilities you carry.

The first thing you can start to do is notice if and when you're holding your breath. If you simply start tuning in to how you're breathing when you're providing care to another, you're off to a great beginning. At first you may be surprised at how much you catch yourself grimacing or holding your breath through the difficult tasks of caregiving. Simply invite opportunities to allow mindful breathing into each experience. That in and of itself is a mindfulness practice.

In addition to mindful breathing, gently notice your thoughts when you're actively providing care, as well as when you're thinking about the care you have to provide. Notice how much you're worrying about what's to come. You might find it helpful to integrate the practices that have been shared in this chapter, as well as previous chapters, when you notice worry, tension, or anxiety in your mind or body. You can bring present-moment activities awareness to your caregiving activities, such as preparing food, bathing, transporting, or simply being with your loved one.

The reduced stress that may result from integrating this practice in your caregiving responsibilities may translate into your loved one's perceptions of being cared for and feeling calm and at ease.

PARENT MINDFULLY.

If your responsibilities involve caring for your children, you may want to consider the concept of mindful parenting (Bögels and Restifo 2014). Often what children crave and need most is the intentional focus and care of their parents and loved ones. If you take the time to talk to any parent of a child who is of high school age or on the way to college, what they almost always share is how fast the time has flown. They cannot believe that their child, who was once a little bitty baby, is now emerging into adulthood and on the verge of independence. These parents often remark that they wish they could have slowed down time. They advise parents of young children to cherish the moments, take lots of photos and videos, and spend as much time as possible with their precious young ones.

The concept of mindful parenting relates to this wise advice. Every single moment you're with your children is an opportunity to practice mindfulness. Mindfulness does not always have to involve a fancy cushion, yoga postures, or memorizing the steps to the body scan or the walking meditation. The essence of mindfulness—present-moment, nonjudgmental awareness, and heartfulness with your senses—can be practiced as you engage with your children. Each moment with your children brings an opportunity to practice mindful listening, mindful speech, mindful patience, and loving-kindness. You even have rich opportunities to practice mindful self-compassion when you feel you've been less than perfect as a parent—perhaps you made a mistake, yelled too loudly, set a "bad" example, forgot an important date, or had to miss an important event in your child's life. Bringing self-compassion to yourself can remind you of your own humanity, allow you to forgive yourself, and demonstrate to your children how *they* may practice self-compassion in their own lives. It has been said there are not many better opportunities to practice mindfulness than through mindful parenting. You have plenty of opportunities to practice over and over again—without shame, blame, or guilt.

INTEGRATE INFORMAL PRACTICES AT WORK, DURING ERRANDS, OR WHEREVER YOU GO.

The moral of this chapter is that mindfulness can be practiced anywhere you go and at any time. The time is almost always right for some form of mindfulness practice. The formal practices, such as the body scan, sitting meditation, mindful walking, loving-kindness meditation, and mindful yoga require more dedicated space, time, or focus because they are, well, formal. However, *informal* mindfulness practice is always just a breath away. When you're washing the dishes, you can be mindfully aware of how the warm, soapy dishwater touches your hands. When you're cleaning your house, you can practice mindful gratitude for all the things you possess and the blessing of having a roof over your head. When you're doing laundry, you can practice intentional mindful awareness and gratitude for each item as it goes into the wash, comes out of the warmth of the dryer, and gets folded and put away with care. When you're on hold as you're making a medical appointment, booking a hotel room, or paying a bill, listening to the soft music can be an opportunity to check in with your body and your breath with mindful intention. Instead of approaching these experiences with stress or dread, you can actually de-stress when you bring an intention of informal mindfulness practice. You may be surprised to find how many experiences during your waking moments bring opportunity to breathe, show compassion, and experience connection to others with loving-kindness.

Conclusion

This chapter was written to fill your toolkit and support your overall success in living with joy and well-being. With time, you can practice mindfulness in *everything* you do. These tips can help:

● Integrate formal mindfulness practice with just one to two minutes at a time.

● Practice mindfulness during everyday activities, like washing dishes, cleaning the house, or doing the laundry.

● Practice mindfulness of sound—engage in the present movement of birdsongs, yard equipment, or other sounds.

● Practice mindfulness when providing care to children or other loved ones.

● Practice mindfulness when you're listening to others talk.

● Practice mindfulness when you're speaking to others.

● Practice mindful walking whenever you walk from place to place.

● Practice mindful gratitude when people show you patience or kindness.

May you continue to enjoy this journey to help you cope with stress mindfully and with self-compassion.

~Peace~

CHAPTER 8

Connect with Nature and Art

When it comes to mindfulness practice—being in and appreciating the present moment, without judgment and with heartfulness—there are two resources that continuously provide rich opportunities to be reflective and at peace. Spending time with nature and immersing yourself in various forms of art can yield opportunities for a mind-body connection that enhances the depth of your journey to self-care, wholeness, and healing (Myers 1988). As we learned through engaging with the leaves on the stream meditation practice in Chapter 7, emotional states and physical sensations can be transformed through mindful presence with nature. The same is true of engaging with the arts.

Engaging in nature and the arts involves opportunities to have sensory experiences that can simultaneously be both simple and complex. Nature and the arts provide low-cost ways to observe, reflect, and experience your surroundings that can lower stress and connect you to the core of who you are, with stillness. Although connecting with certain forms of nature or the arts can provide universally positive experiences, you also may have preferences for what generates optimal joy and respite for yourself. In this chapter, you will have the opportunity to consider what experiences of nature and the arts may work most ideally and beneficially to enhance your emotional and physical well-being.

Connecting with the Arts

Similar to nature, the brilliance of human-generated artistic expression provides opportunities for mindful awareness. Products of art include drawings, photographs, paintings, instrumental music, song lyrics, poetry, choreography, pottery, fashion, and even architecture. These awe-inspiring artistic expressions are literally at your fingertips. The diversity of the arts can provide you with the ability to select experiences that resonate with your spirit in ways that can enhance your emotional and physical well-being.

Art Museum Experiences

Many cities—large or small—have art museums or galleries awaiting your arrival. Museums provide formal and informal opportunities to engage with various types of artistic expressions, including photography, paintings, drawings, and sculpture. Informal experiences with museums can include day trips to engage with special exhibits or pieces of art. Perhaps you will be inspired by the quiet observation of artistic pieces as you meander through galleries and curated hallways.

Formal art museum experiences may include workshops or seminars with art educators. One particular art museum experience is referred to as "close looking" or "visual thinking" (Yenawine and Miller 2014). During these intentional group-based activities, museum visitors are encouraged to first mindfully and silently take in works of art, and then engage in compassion-generating reflective conversations in response to three formal questions: "What is going on in this work of art?" "What do you see that makes you say that?" "What more can we find?" Although these three questions are simple and unassuming, the conversations and reflections that are generated can have immense value and positive outcomes. Research has shown that engagement in close looking or visual thinking can improve critical thinking, empathy, and understanding of self and others, as well as encouraging compassionate communication with a deeper ability to listen and speak effectively. When moderated effectively by an experienced facilitator, engagement in visual thinking strategies and other arts-based practices can also yield reductions in automatic thinking, impatience, and assumptions or bias about others (Gaufberg and Williams 2011; Slavin, Williams, and Zimmermann 2023; Williams and Zimmermann 2020). Although these practices were designed to take place in museums, pandemic-related adaptations have made it possible to engage in these activities in virtual spaces. Most large museums even share their gallery treasures via websites to remove barriers to engagement.

Artistic Mindful Movement

Mindful movement may involve personal or observed experiences with dance. Perhaps you could consider taking in a performance at a cultural center or theater at locations that are in close proximity to your home. You might consider enrolling in a local dance class. Whether you're a beginner or advanced, the opportunity to purposefully move your body rhythmically to the sounds of music can enhance self-awareness, body wisdom, and overall health. In previous research that involved interviews with Black men and women who were experienced mindfulness practitioners, they were asked about activities in Black or African American culture that involved mindfulness (Woods-Giscombé and Gaylord 2014). Participants shared that dancing was a mindfulness activity. One said:

> "When you're dancing, you're in the present. There's nothing else going on."

Expressions were shared regarding the mind-body connection of dance, including the oneness with the music and the natural and satisfying movements of the body that provided stress relief and the release of tension and concerns.

How could you integrate more mindful movement or opportunities to observe or engage in dance in your everyday life? If your geographic location limits your involvement with these activities in person, consider engaging with artistic expressions via television or the internet. Truly consider how you may have fun with artistic mindful movement. You might even try classes or activities provided via videoconference.

Does fingerpainting sound too messy to you, or does this activity sound like an interesting opportunity to integrate mindfulness and creativity? What about photography? Baking or other culinary arts? Even gardening could be considered an artistic endeavor—especially if you use what you grow to develop a culinary work of art.

The activation of sensory experiences such as touching, seeing, smelling, and hearing can stimulate positive emotions that have been dampened by chronic exposure to stress or trauma. Large universities and smaller community colleges provide opportunities for you to create your own artistic expressions through painting, drawing, photography, or clay work. The arts also include sewing, knitting, and quilting— additional practices identified in research as mindfulness based (Woods-Giscombé and Gaylord 2014).

Mindfulness Through Music

You may be someone who enjoys live music. When was the last time you took in a concert? If jazz is your thing, maybe you can schedule an outing to a jazz event with your friends. Perhaps outdoor concerts, symphony concerts, or even the opera appeal to you. Did you know that an array of opportunities is right at your doorstep? Even your local high school choral or orchestra concert may be just what suits your needs.

Have you considered learning how to play an instrument? Or perhaps you played an instrument as a child and are willing to consider reviving your foregone talents. Perhaps an African drumming class sounds appealing to you. One research participant mentioned that mindfulness meditation reminded her of African cultural practices, including communal rituals. These activities could include singing or playing instruments, "something that is passed down that you can do together…that's important to do as part of life." This participant also mentioned the use of meditative drumming and other forms of music that are used therapeutically. Drumming and dancing have been shown in research to help with stress management and perceptions of wellness and quality of life in ways that are similar to other formal practices of mindfulness (Vinesett et al. 2017). Maybe you've always wanted to learn to play the piano or you want to start with a keyboard or a recorder. No instrument is too minor or inconsequential regarding its potential healing benefits—perhaps the tambourine or the cymbals can serve as your entry to musical creativity.

Connecting with Nature

There are so many opportunities to engage with nature mindfully. Have you ever stepped outside and noticed how the gentle breeze caresses your cheek? Perhaps the sound of the wind is a welcome opportunity to remember to allow your breath to flow in and out without straining. Observing the gentle bend of the leaves on tree limbs as they move from side to side can remind us to be nimble in moments of distress. Perhaps even an observation of bees visiting the interior of a colorful blossom can bring an opportunity for mindful pause and wonderment.

Have you ever noticed the intentional movement of an insect on a sidewalk, moving slowly and steadily toward its destination? At night, the on-and-off flicker of light from a firefly against the darkness of the sky may bring awe and inspiration. The smell of fresh-cut grass on a hot summer day can provide an opportunity for present-moment appreciation. Even a cloudy day can be approached with curiosity. As the clouds move—without hurry or anxiety—across the backdrop of the blue sky, they may form magnificent shapes that inspire your imagination and admiration.

When you consider how connecting with nature may yield mindful awareness, perhaps you envision a relaxing beach scene. Palm trees may be waving from side to side, surrounded by floral bushes, acres of golden sand, and blue waves of the ocean as far as the eye can see. Each wave moving in and out toward the shore can be an opportunity for mindful breathing with awareness—with nothing else to do and nowhere else to go but to be fully present and surrounded by both visual and auditory sensations. The sound of crashing waves can yield a peaceful presence and appreciation for the ability to *just be*. This scene may be further enhanced by views of seabirds soaring in the sky—rising to heights and then dipping and diving into cool ocean waters for a meal. The circle of life continues.

Although walking upright on the shore may be a perfect opportunity for mindfulness, you might also choose to integrate mindful movement as you bend to select seashells that are particularly attractive to you. Perhaps you're drawn to the glistening white shells that sparkle on the ground, or you may be captivated by the smooth dark shells that stand out from their background of beige and gold sand. The act of identifying and picking up shells is also an opportunity for mindful presence. You may notice small sea crabs that scurry into coastal holes leading to their burrows. The warmth of the sun on your face may be energizing for you. The sea mist carried by the ocean breeze might provide a sense of uplift and joy.

While tranquil to many, the beach is not the only opportunity for mindful presence with nature. In your own backyard, on your front porch, or on neighborhood streets you may be fascinated with the activities of nature. Perhaps you're enchanted by the sounds of thunder before a storm, the startling flash of lightning in the sky, the gentle or dramatic sounds of rain pelting the ground, or the sweet smell of the air after a cleansing rainfall. You may tune in to the morning songs of birds outside your window or the conversations of crickets on a warm summer evening.

Perhaps the calming fall of winter's snow brings a sense of joy to your spirit. The quietness as snow drifts to the ground may be an opportunity for you to engage in silent stillness. Your observation of snow-birds making trails in the white fluffy substance may renew hope and delight. The outdoor coldness is refreshing, while also yielding an appreciation for the warmth of indoors. Perhaps the crackling of an outdoor firepit or living room fireplace is the promise of toasty coziness after a cold outdoor experience.

Moment-to-moment presence with the celestial bodies may also provide occasions for mindful renewal. The promise of the sunrise on the horizon at dawn. The sky transitioning from darkness to light. Similarly, the setting of the sun in the evening and the appearance of the moon and the stars provide awe-inspiring awareness of the known and the unknown of the universe. You may be reminded that you're part of a larger purpose and encouraged to rise above the minute details or challenges of life that are inevitable, yet need not be the focus of your existence.

The natural world provides so many opportunities for discovery and wholeness. The shade of the forest during a quiet, autumn walk, or the crunch of fallen leaves of golden and reddish hue under your feet allow the sounds of your thoughts to gently dissipate. You may observe birds' nests, busy squirrels, or meticulously created spider webs reflecting the light of the sun penetrating through the trees. Some of the things you experience in nature may be somewhat disturbing or even scary. For instance, if you're fearful of spiders, coming upon a large spider web may be alarming at first. What if you consider the grandeur of this creation and the wisdom of how the web supports the spider's survival? Birds pecking at worms after a morning rain could seem uncomfortable to you at first glance, but you might remind yourself that the birds are simply eating their breakfast. As you take in these nature scenes, you realize they all have purpose and intention.

Time for Practice: Mountain Meditation

As you consider opportunities to connect with nature in ways that are mindful and supportive of your well-being, *mountain meditation* can be a helpful practice to add to your meditation toolkit.

This meditation can be done just about anywhere that you can be in uninterrupted stillness for as long as you have time to practice. You can do mountain meditation indoors or outside in nature. Of course, you can use a real mountain to guide your practice. However, all you really need is your mind and your breath.

Step-by-Step Guidance for the Mountain Meditation

Begin by giving yourself a few moments of pause. Allow yourself to find an intentional connection with your breath. Perhaps allowing your eyes to relax from taking in visual stimulation. Allow your eyelids to lower, with your eyes gently open and not focused on any particular view, or you may allow your eyes to close.

Next, become aware of your breathing—perhaps the rise and fall of your chest and any tightness in your chest area. As you breathe in and out, allow what feels tight or heavy to lighten and expand. Bringing your awareness from your chest area to the rising and falling of your belly.

Noticing the surface that is supporting your weight and allowing yourself to be supported without holding on to any tension in your hips or lower body. Noticing your face and allowing the area below your cheekbones to drop a bit, releasing any tension from your face. Perhaps even allowing space between your upper and lower teeth. Gently allowing your tongue to relax, your forehead to soften, and your throat to become supple. You may also bring awareness to the sides of your neck as you follow the breath down to your shoulders, allowing them to lower—arms to soften and hands to rest either in your lap or at your sides. With your feet becoming more grounded and supported by the surface beneath them. With awareness of your whole, living, and breathing body—inhaling and exhaling at your own pace—with nothing to do and nowhere to be other than just where you are at this moment. Perhaps even allowing a gentle smile on your face.

Now allowing an image of a mountain to come to your mind's eye. No pushing or rushing this image to arrive, but gently inviting a scene of a mountain into your consciousness. The mountain that is coming to your awareness may be a mountain you've seen before or one you've only imagined. Take a few moments to take in your mountain. Perhaps it's a tall green mountain covered with grass and trees with a sharp peak. Maybe your mountain stands out in a series of mountains, and it has a softer peak covered by snow. Or maybe the mountain you're envisioning is a rocky one with jagged edges. Whatever image is coming into your view, simply take a few moments to be with that mountain—allowing its image to sharpen in your mind's eye. The peak or series of peaks at the top of the mountain, the sides or slopes of the mountain, and the base of the mountain connecting it to the solid earth. The mountain may appear to be strong, powerful, stately, unmoving, grounded, yet upright.

As you take in the mountain, with awareness of your breath and your own body, you might see that you're much like the mountain. With your head as the lofty peak, your shoulders and arms like the slopes and sides of the mountain, and your seat like the solid mountain base. You may notice your upright posture, allowing you to be as strong, powerful, stately, unmoving, and grounded as the mountain.

As you sit like a living, breathing mountain, bring to your awareness the various experiences that come to visit the mountain. At times, rain may fall on the mountain. There may be other days when the mountain is covered in clouds or fog, and it's not as easy to see the mountain's peak or its sharp or gentle slopes. Nevertheless, the essence of the mountain does not change. Despite what is going on around or on the mountain, its rootedness, its integrity, its stateliness, and its uplift don't change.

Around the mountain, the heat of summer brings brightness, yet aridness and drought. The coolness of fall brings bright, bold colors, followed by opportunities for rest. The cold of winter brings snow, wind, and ice, as well as coziness and reflection. The promise of spring brings rebirth, hope, birdsongs, and new opportunities for growth. As seasons change, what appears on the surface of the mountain may change. Yet, underneath it all, the mountain continues to be grounded—through calmness and turbulence. From dawn to dusk, from the height of the sun at noon to the height of the moon at night.

Others have their own personal relationship with the mountain. People see the mountain up close with familiarity, or from afar with awe. No matter how close to or distant from the mountain others are, they experience it with unawareness of all that the mountain is experiencing. However, the mountain often serves as a source of inspiration. For some, the mountain may even provide shade from the sun, or a sense of central location or landmark of familiarity that helps others from feeling lost. The mountain may even have caves or tall trees that serve as a shield from unknown or unexpected danger—providing safety and protection. Yet sometimes the mountain may be a source of frustration or disappointment when clouds, fog, or storms keep it from being accessible or in clear view.

Despite others' experiences of the mountain and despite what is going on around the mountain, despite its season or the current experiences of weather, the mountain continues to *be*—uplifted, unmoving, grounded, stately, and powerful.

As you take in the fullness of the mountain, as well as its experiences with the natural world and with others—consider how you're just like the mountain. Despite it all, despite the weather or season, despite who comes to see the mountain, who needs the mountain, who hopes to be shielded by the mountain, or who is inspired (or not) by the mountain—despite stress or strain, pain or joy—the beauty and the essence of the mountain continues to endure.

Mountain meditation can be a reminder of these qualities that you possess as often as you choose to practice. Like other qualities in nature and the arts, mountains have a lot to teach us, if we allow them to do so.

Time for Reflection

It may be helpful to journal your responses to these questions:

→ What feelings and thoughts came to the forefront as you engaged in the mountain meditation?

→ What types of "weathering" have you experienced in ways similar to the experiences of the mountain?

→ In what ways have you endured changes in seasons or external circumstances in your life?

→ How have you stayed in touch with the core of who you are despite changes that may have occurred all around you?

→ What characteristics of mountains can you use to thrive in the midst of the changing (and sometimes unsettling) circumstances around you?

Conclusion

There are boundless opportunities through nature and the arts. It may be helpful to take some time to consider what thoughts, feelings, and emotions came up for you as you read this chapter. As your senses have opportunities to take in the awe-inspiring stimulation of nature and the arts, you possess new and unpredictable opportunities—day after day— to practice the seven pillars of mindfulness including acceptance, beginner's mind, nonjudgment, letting go, patience, trust, and non-striving. Accepting the mighty expressions of art and nature as they are, from moment to moment and from breath to breath, provides resources to support you as you manage stress and build your coping toolkit. May you continue to be well on your way along your journey to health and well-being.

~Peace~

CHAPTER 9

Mindfully Relate to Family and Friends

There are few things more special than the bonds of family and friends. When I was writing this chapter, I was a bystander at the beach, observing an outdoor wedding ceremony. The people were all total strangers to me, but I could sense the love and affection between the newlyweds and their loved ones. The commitment that these two people were making to one another had brought together family and friends. I could sense that the other bystanders around the couple and their loved ones also felt this sacred energy, as they watched in silence and with respect for this special, unifying event.

The couple's family and friends witnessed the vows and publicly affirmed their willingness to support and uplift the couple "through sickness and through health." I cannot think of many things more heartful than occasions such as this. Observing the wedding brought tears to my eyes.

However, it's also true that as beautiful, loving, and sacred as familial bonds can be, these bonds also can bring their own share of challenges. There may be unexpected twists and turns in any relationship. For example, as a couple vows to come together as one, they are also encouraged to cherish and respect each other's individuality and unique qualities. In your case, despite the support and affection that relationships bring, you might also find that your partner and other family members may have a difficult time accepting your personal nuances and quirks. They are closest to you, and they more easily see the specific activities and ebbs and flows of your daily life. Family members and friends are also affected when you decide to make changes in your life.

Resistance to or concerns about the changes you're making might be particularly evident if your loved ones perceive you as the core or the backbone of your family. Your family and friends may be thrown off balance when you change your routine, even when the changes are positive. Your existence may be a crucial foundation for their lives and experiences. If you make changes in your everyday habits, then your family members, friends, and loved ones feel this shift directly in their lives. They may applaud your healthy changes, but the modifications you've made to your life might also be destabilizing for them. Your loved ones may wonder, *If she makes changes in her life, what's going to happen to me?*

These are the very questions that may cause you to delay prioritizing your personal health and well-being. You may fear that caring for yourself is selfish and will mean that you have less time and energy to help those loved ones who need you. Although you may find value and purpose in being there to help them, potential guilt related to feeling like you're not doing enough for your loved ones may impede your ability to make sustainable changes to improve your emotional and physical wellness.

For example, how many times have you made plans to take a morning walk, and just when you're about to be out the door, you get a call or text from a family member who needs your help or advice? How many times have you tried to set routines to go to the gym in the evening, but work projects, committee meetings, or a child's rehearsal end up taking precedence? What about those times when you committed to eating healthier, then along came your family's push to eat less healthy meals? You wound up eating tasty traditional foods that challenged your healthy goals for your waistline and your arteries. Maybe you've even made a decision that getting more sleep is a priority, but your promises to provide last-minute edits, alterations, or assistance on other unexpected projects challenge your goals to put your health and well-being first.

Is your practice changing how you think? Is your new mindful way of living changing how you communicate? Are you finding that you have new preferences related to how you eat, where you like to go, or even who you like to be around? Perhaps you're seeking more peace in your life, and that is starting to mean letting go of people, places, and things that haven't served you well—people, places, and things that possibly caused you emotional stress or strain. Prior to your mindfulness practice, perhaps you weren't yet aware that you had *choices* to create new healthy situations for yourself independent of other cultural or familial patterns and traditions you felt the need to uphold.

However, as healthy as your new choices may be, change is not always easy. Change (even if it's to advance your well-being) can cause uncertainty, isolation, and loneliness. You've started new habits, behaviors, and ways of thinking that may be different from those of your family members, loved ones, and friends. The results of this may at times feel like too much. Giving up familiarity or spending less time with people who are in your social circle may not feel like it's worth the potential benefits of improving other aspects of your health. Perhaps you're afraid of or concerned about the potential impact on your social life and relationships with loved ones. These concerns or fears can be a deterrent to sustaining healthy changes in your habits or overall lifestyle.

It's also possible that your family members or loved ones don't quite understand this new practice of meditation that you've incorporated into your life. Mindfulness meditation may be a new concept for them. They may even wonder if you've changed your religion. In fact, their reactions may cause you to feel conflicted between your new meditation practice and the religious beliefs you may have learned about and practiced since you were a child.

Do any of these ideas and feelings resonate with you? As you reflect on the challenges you experience with sustaining new mindfulness-based healthy habits, what barriers can you identify? What fears do you have that are related to change? And how might those barriers or fears be addressed?

One of the easiest potential challenges related to your new mindfulness meditation practice to address is the issue related to religion or spirituality. Mindfulness is *not* a religion. Your practice of mindfulness does not have to conflict with your personal, familial, or cultural religious beliefs or practices. Mindfulness (by definition) is simply paying attention, on purpose, without judgment, and with heartfulness (Kabat-Zinn 2013). Mindfulness helps you develop awareness of yourself, your feelings, your thoughts, your situations, and your relationships with others—but practicing mindfulness does not have to mean changing your religion. It does not have to conflict with your previous spiritual practices. In fact, some women in research studies I've led shared that practicing mindfulness deepened their personal religious practices. More specifically, women have shared that mindfulness practice has helped them be more attentive during religious ceremonies, such as church services. Many also shared that their mindfulness practice helped them deepen their prayer practice because they had become better able to stay focused during their prayers. Mindfulness also enhanced their ability to demonstrate faithfulness; they were less worried, scattered, or anxious because of the deeper awareness of their thoughts and the effect of their thoughts on their emotions generated through mindfulness practice.

There are many images of meditation in the media, including on television or in print, that may cause your loved ones to question if your new practices are congruent or in conflict with your religion. Meditation or yoga postures, symbols, attire, or cultural references may lead to some of these concerns. Consider how you might communicate with your loved ones to share more about why you've chosen to practice mindfulness, the definition of mindfulness, and how it benefits you. Your mindfulness practice might even help you with skillfully communicating this information to your loved ones. These conversations may relieve any concerns they have about mindfulness practice.

You might even gently invite your loved ones to practice mindfulness with you. Perhaps engaging in mindful eating, walking meditation, body scan meditation, or even loving-kindness meditation may be excellent introductions to mindfulness for your loved ones. They might understand more about what mindfulness is. They may even notice the personal benefits of mindfulness for themselves. Your gentle and compassionate ways of helping them understand mindfulness may even result in your having a new mindfulness meditation partner. It's truly possible that the more they know, the less likely they are to resist your interest in cultivating more mindfulness in your life or even in your household and everyday existence. As a result, your relationships might even be strengthened in the long run.

You can use your mindfulness to address the potential challenges described in this chapter. Approaching their concerns with compassion and empathy may yield positive benefits that go beyond their concerns about mindfulness. Additionally, as you continue to prioritize your wellness, your family members and loved ones may eventually be inspired by what they see you *do* versus what they hear you *say*. Witnessing you as a more grounded, joyful, physically and emotionally healthy person may cause them to want to engage themselves more in the new ways of life you've adopted. They may even see that the healthier you are, the more you're able to show up for them in ways that are optimally healthy and whole.

Time for Practice: Kinship Connection Meditation

Despite all the encouragement you're receiving in this book, you may continue to have concerns that your new commitment to prioritizing self-care could have negative consequences. Perhaps you continue to fear that focusing on self-care is selfish and it will mean (or be perceived by others) that you're somehow abandoning your responsibilities to be there for your family members and friends. You may even continue to be concerned that the ways you'll change with regard to new healthy behaviors and your new healthy mindset will somehow isolate you from your loved ones. Perhaps they have noticed how you're already changing, and you can sense discomfort or concern in them. Maybe your family members and friends are cheering you along on your journey, yet they have remarked that, although your lifestyle changes work for you, they don't seem achievable to them. Or maybe some of them have begun to join you, and you want to find ways to continue to sustain this engagement in healthy habits as a circle of family members or friends.

The *kinship connection meditation* is an extension of the loving-kindness meditation practice that may help keep you inspired and encouraged regarding the potential power and benefits of continuing to prioritize your personal wellness. As you develop new habits, you're not the only person who will experience benefits. Everyone else in your midst will have the potential to experience the value of prioritizing wellness. As you learn new ways to respond to stress and challenges in your life, others may also develop coping strategies that help interrupt the connections between stress and undesirable health outcomes.

The kinship connection meditation allows you to bring your circle of loved ones into this experience—not just the loved ones you see and spend time with on a regular basis, but also your loved ones who may have passed along, including those from previous generations like grandparents, aunts, uncles, and others you may never even have met.

Step-by-Step Guidance
for the Kinship Connection Meditation

You can begin this meditation with an intention for presence and regard for the sacred connections of family and friends. It will be helpful to gather items essential to this practice ahead of time. Start with a collection of photographs of your family members and friends. Various types of photos may be used; including group photos, family portraits, posed pictures, active photos, or headshots. Although you may be used to storing such pictures on your phone or tablet, it will be helpful to print out your loved ones' photos for this meditation practice. Try to have as many people as possible represented. It may be helpful to have these photographs framed, but that is not a requirement.

Once you have the photos ready, place them on a large table or counter in no particular order, and take a seat. As you're sitting, allow yourself to experience a mindful presence with awareness of your physical body and what you're feeling emotionally about engaging in this practice. While remaining open to the range of emotions this experience might generate, intentionally invite emotions of love, openheartedness, and the generosity of compassion— for yourself and for others—and allow the most loving place in your heart to lead you in this experience.

Allow time for a gentle scan of your body from head to face, to neck to chest, to shoulders, belly, back, hip, thighs, knees, legs, ankles, feet, and toes. Allowing the breath to move through your body at your own pace, with a sense of flow and ease. Noticing your eyes resting in their sockets, your ears open for sounds, and your hands soft, supple, and at rest at your sides or on your lap. Noticing your chest or belly rise and fall with exhalation and inhalation. Now bring a more pronounced, focused attention to your hands. If your eyes are closed or downcast, allow them to open or look up and take in the sight of the photos.

One by one, begin to touch each photo—generating love and affection for the people captured in the images. Holding each loved one with reverence and extending the wishes of loving-kindness—one by one. May you be well, may you be at peace, may you have comfort, may you be loved. Sharing these wishes with each loved one in the photo. Taking as much time as you need with a connection of your heart to theirs. Wishing as much for them as you're hoping for yourself on this wellness journey. May you be free from stress, may you overcome challenges, may you experience joy and tranquility, and may you be healthy. Repeating these or similar phrases with each person, and then repeating the same back to yourself. May I be well, may I be at peace, may I have comfort, may I be loved. May I be free from stress, may I overcome my challenges, may I experience joy and tranquility, and may I be healthy.

If you have photos of ancestors who are no longer on this earth, you may find it strange to be sending them these present-moment wishes, yet these may be the most important sentiments to share. As you recall, you may have received messages from your mothers, fathers, grandmothers, grandfathers, aunts, or uncles that influence your relationships to stress, rest, self-care, and wellness. In some way, your wellness journey is connected to their experiences. Sharing these wishes with departed loved ones may (in love) help shift or release the experiences in their lives that continue to serve as challenges in yours. Sharing the same sentiments with those departed loved ones through intentional presence with their photos. May you be well, may you be at peace, may you have comfort, may you be loved. May you be free from stress, may you overcome challenges, may you experience joy and tranquility, and may you be healthy. You may even add: May your dreams come true, may you be all that you hoped for, and may you be honored through the lives of your children and loved ones.

Take time to notice the thoughts and emotions that may be with you during this meditation. Acknowledging what you're feeling and allowing your breath to continue to flow. Checking in with your heart and body, releasing tension that may arise—gently through exhalation. Continuing to breathe in your intentions of wellness and love.

You may want to arrange the photos as you're sharing the wishes of loving-kindness, creating a photo display table that you can easily visit when you want to repeat this practice or simply spend time with these loved ones via their photographs. If your religion or spirituality honors the practice of prayer, you can choose to extend prayers for yourself and for your loved ones during this time. You can also allow yourself to receive the same loving-kindness wishes that you've offered to your loved ones. Receive your loved ones sharing those messages with you. Allow yourself space to breathe in and breathe out as you allow the beauty, love, and support of these messages to wash over your entire being. With gratitude, accept the positive nature in which you're giving and receiving as part of this kinship connection meditation.

If there are loved ones that you'd like to honor through this practice, but you don't have photos of them, there are a couple of things you can do. You can bring items that remind you of those individuals, or you can simply write their names on a piece of paper and see them in your imagination. Once you have the items or names, you can repeat the same phrases of loving-kindness or extend similar prayers, as you would have if you had their photos.

Once you become familiar with the guidance for engaging in this practice, feel free to make it your own. Do what comes instinctually to you as you spend time sharing love and warm messages with yourself and your loved ones. The practice of kinship connection is meant to acknowledge the seen and unseen bonds you have with your loved ones, recognizing that your journey is in many ways connected to their journeys, and that whether or not they are where you are with prioritizing wellness, they can be part of your wellness journey.

In doing this practice, you're granting *yourself* permission to retain what is helpful and healthful and release what is not without turning your back on your loved ones, on their customs, beliefs, or habits. By engulfing them with intentions for wellness, you *may be* in some way influencing the trajectory of their wellness journey through conscious prioritization of your own personal wellness. This gift may not only benefit you but others as well.

Time for Reflection

As you consider the lifestyle changes you're making to improve your emotional and physical health, please reflect upon how these changes are impacting your family, friends, and loved ones. As you consider these questions, it may be helpful to journal what comes up for you.

→ How have your family, friends, and loved ones responded to your changes?

→ In what ways have they shown curiosity about the new things you're doing?

→ In what ways have they shown resistance to the new things you're doing?

→ In what ways have they been supportive?

→ How have your new habits changed the way you communicate with them?

→ How might your attention to self-care be a positive influence for them?

→ What were the negative effects of this attention?

→ In what ways have you limited your progress as a result of concerns about how your family or friends will react or have reacted?

→ Based on your reflections, what comes up for you as important action steps?

→ How can you care about your family members and friends without carrying the load of their concerns and challenges?

→ How can you simultaneously love and care for them, while loving and caring for yourself in meaningful ways?

Perhaps you're finding it helpful to journal your responses to these questions. It may even be valuable to discuss them with a trusted and supportive person in your life. Remember that as you change, your family and friends will respond to this change. Change can be good. You *can* navigate this change mindfully, and you can continue to move forward on your journey to be healthy, happy, and whole!

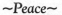

~Peace~

CHAPTER 10

Move into Your New Future of Wellness

As the saying goes, "You've come a long way, baby." It's safe to say that you picked up this book for the first time in a different place, emotionally and physically, than you are now. Some force caused you to be attracted to this book. Perhaps you were attracted to its title. You may have been intrigued by the colorful cover. Perhaps a friend recommended the book. You may have learned about it on social media, on a news show, in your favorite magazine, or on the shelf in your local bookstore.

You may have been struggling for a long time, and possibly silently, with feelings of distress and even hopelessness as you carried burdens that no one knew you were carrying. You may have been feeling stress, anxiety, sleeplessness, or even sadness. You may have been at a place of wondering if experiencing a life of joy could possibly be in your future. You may have been attracted to this book because you were experiencing physical symptoms of distress, such as headaches, unexplained sickness, chronic body pain, or physical exhaustion and burnout. Whatever your reason for reading the first word of this book, I'm grateful that you stayed with it to arrive at this final chapter.

Through engaging with the previous nine chapters, you've gained so much information. Chapter 1 introduced you to the links between stress, coping, and the Superwoman Schema in Black women. You learned about stress and how it contributes to disproportionately high

rates of chronic health conditions in Black women. You had an opportunity to think about your own health and well-being, as well as the
health and well-being of other Black women in your life (your mother,
your grandmothers, your sister, and your friends). With information
about the effects of stress on physical, emotional, and behavioral processes that influence health, you were able to consider how ways of
coping with stress may be helpful, as well as harmful. You read quotes
and anecdotes from Black women about how the Superwoman Schema
characteristics may develop, how they may be helpful or adaptive, and
how they may be harmful. Information from research was provided
regarding evidence of the potential protective nature of the Superwoman
Schema. This may have been the first time you were invited to consider
whether stress-related health problems are avoidable. You were introduced to the brief breathing space meditation as an initial step to taking
a break from stress and interrupting the effects of stress on your mental
and physical well-being.

The next five chapters provided deeper content on the characteristics of the Superwoman Schema, and how each may operate in women's
lives, including yours. In Chapter 2, you learned about the Superwoman
Schema concept of being strong no matter what. You took the opportunity to reflect on your own personal definition of strength, and you
considered the ways in which strength contributes to and limits your
goals of being healthy and happy. As part of your opportunity to reflect
on how the first Superwoman Schema characteristic of strength operates in your life, you were introduced to sitting meditation as a foundational meditation practice.

In Chapter 3, you considered the Superwoman Schema concept of
suppressing your emotions. You had the opportunity to define what it
means when Black women are encouraged to uphold the idea of not
showing emotions, and you considered your own personal definitions
and experiences with emotional suppression, including when it serves
you and when it hinders you. You learned about adaptive or healthy

strategies for expressing and releasing emotions for psychological and physical well-being. You were introduced to the body scan meditation and encouraged to reflect upon your own personal mind-body connection to promote self-wisdom and wellness.

In Chapter 4, you were invited to consider how the third Superwoman Schema characteristic may operate in your life. You were provided with space to reflect upon how you may "resist being vulnerable or depending on others for help." A working definition of this characteristic was provided, and you reflected on your own personal definition of resistance to being vulnerable and resistance to depending on others. You learned about strategies for optimally using this characteristic when it may be adaptive or helpful, as well as strategies for finding ways to allow this characteristic to exist within yourself for self-protective purposes, while also considering the benefits of allowing trusted others to provide help and support to you. The mutual health benefits of interconnection/social connection were covered in this chapter with guidance for you to develop strategies to minimize emotional suppression or self-reliance behaviors that may be harmful to your emotional or physical health. You were introduced to wise heartfulness meditation and encouraged to find ways to integrate this practice into your life.

In Chapter 5, you explored the fourth Superwoman Schema characteristic, being motivated to succeed despite limited resources. You were invited to consider how this characteristic operates in your personal and professional life and the factors that may have contributed to its development. A working definition of this characteristic was provided, and you were invited to reflect on your own personal definition of this characteristic as you read through anecdotes of characters shared in the chapter, including examples of how women beat the odds despite limited resources. You also were invited to consider your own perceptions of what it means to have limited resources, as well as strategies for seeing yourself as resourceful, and strategies for creating a worldview of resources as boundless and ever-present. In this chapter, you were introduced to breathing space meditation and mindful movement, including walking meditation and mindful stretching. You were invited to consider how you might integrate these practices more regularly in your life.

In Chapter 6, you were introduced to the fifth Superwoman Schema characteristic: prioritizing caregiving over self-care. You had the opportunity to reflect on the ways that you may be prioritizing the needs of others over your own needs. You also reflected on barriers to self-care (for example, guilt, stigma, models from other women, expectations from loved ones, personal definitions of what it means to be a caring, supportive woman). You were encouraged to consider that you don't have to stop engaging in caregiving activities. Instead, you were invited to perceive self-care as philanthropic and a conduit toward making optimal contributions of your personal resources and abilities to your family, community, or workplace. You were strongly encouraged to see self-care as nonnegotiable, and you read examples of women who have successfully integrated self-care activities into their lives. You created an action plan for self-care practices that are congruent with your values and feasible for your lifestyle. In addition, you were encouraged to engage in loving-kindness meditation as a way to generate more kindness and compassion for yourself—as well as for others—in ways that don't deplete you, or cause you harm emotionally or physically.

In Chapter 7, we acknowledged the challenges related to creating new habits that enable you to integrate mindfulness and self-care practices into your everyday life. You were invited to identify the meditation practices that you prefer the most. You were also encouraged to identify barriers and facilitators to your engagement in regular, daily mindfulness practice. You learned strategies to help you identify, prioritize, and schedule additional creative, reflective practices to generate mindfulness, self-compassion, and self-care. Tips for practicing mindfulness in the morning and at night were shared, as well as tips for mindful parenting, mindfulness at work, and mindfulness while on the go. You were also invited to consider ways that you might expand your self-care toolkit by integrating more mindfulness and self-care/self-compassion practices into your life.

In Chapter 8, you were invited to reflect upon ways to deepen your commitment to self-care and healing through connecting with nature and the arts. You were encouraged to engage with sensory experiences during activities such as stargazing; weather-related events, such as rain or snowfall; walking on nature trails; noticing the characteristics of the seasonal changes (winter, spring, summer, or fall); bird-watching and listening to birdcalls; and observations of natural bodies of water, such as lakes, ponds, streams, rivers, or oceans. You were also encouraged to engage in experiences with the arts, including visual, dance, musical, and other arts-based practices to enhance the mind-body connection and wellness. You were invited to connect these experiences with nature and the arts to your personal experiences with stress, the Superwoman Schema, and personal coping strategies. You were introduced to the leaves on the stream meditation practice as an approach to deepening your connection to the healing powers of nature.

In Chapter 9, you had the opportunity to think about how your new habits of practicing mindfulness and prioritizing self-care may affect your loved ones, family members, and friends. You were provided with information to normalize their potential responses to the new you. As you considered how you might relate differently to your family members and friends, you were given the opportunity to consider how they might initially resist change. You were encouraged to reflect on how you could help your family understand that although you're changing to become emotionally and physically healthier, you'll still be available to love and care for them—and possibly with more wholeness than ever before. You were also provided with information to help your family understand the concept of mindfulness, including ways to help them understand that your mindfulness practice and your spiritual or religious beliefs don't conflict with one another. You had the opportunity to practice the kinship connection meditation, which may help you experience the power of your new self-care practices for enriching and sustaining the health and well-being of those in your circle of family and friends.

You've committed yourself to wellness and self-care. You now possess a diverse set of tools that you can use on a regular basis to keep yourself happy and healthy. You've discovered joy and fulfillment in *being* simply who you are rather than seeking fulfillment from nonstop *doing*. You no longer feel guilty for prioritizing self-care. You know that caring for yourself is not selfish. Caring for yourself is actually an act of courage and generosity to yourself, as well as to others. You've transformed your trajectory in life. Believe it or not, this radical act of focusing on your well-being is actually an act of service. When people see you practice meditation, and prioritize mindful walking, mindful eating, and mindful resting, the positivity that results from your activities multiplies beneficially in uplifting ways for all those in your midst. The kindness you now habitually show yourself invites others to consider the potential benefits of kindness for themselves. You speak and listen with grounded warmth. The compassion you reflect provides others with examples of how to live compassionately. You walk with a new pep in your step, you glow with an ever-shining light from within. Your actions speak louder than words; or as often stated, you can "show them better than you can tell them."

You've helped open the door so that your family members, friends, and younger generations in your midst can shift the tide of life to the possibilities of wellness. Your new priorities that center around wellness yield blessings and unexpected gifts that can accompany your new mindset and approach to life. The *mindful vision board* practice comprehensively exemplifies this commitment to wholeness, as well as your relationships with others who observe you during your transformation. At this time, you're invited to engage in this potentially powerful practice.

Time for Practice: Mindful Vision Board

The concept of creating vision boards may not be new for you. Perhaps you've been invited to vision board parties at the start of a new year to help you identify and stick to your New Year's resolutions. You may have even created vision boards during strategic planning or personal goal-setting events at work.

Before you begin, gather enough of these items to create at least two vision boards:

- Small or large cardstock, posterboard, or construction paper

- Magazines or catalogs

- Scissors

- Glue or tape

- Markers (optional)

- Glitter or stickers (optional)

- A mindful presence (required ☺)

By now, you may be anticipating one aspect of this practice that is different from other types of vision board activities you may have completed. This mindful vision board practice begins with gentle sitting meditation, body scan meditation, and gentle mindful movement. You may even incorporate some of the other mindfulness practices you've read about in this book, including mindful time with nature and art, loving-kindness, and kinship connection practice. Your experiences with these practices may at this point be so rich that you don't need additional guidance. However, feel free to review the steps for each practice in the previous chapters if you'd like additional guidance. Most of all, find time and an environment that will allow you to focus on the mindful vision board practice without interruption.

Step-by-Step Guidance for the Vision Board

Vision Board #1

As you've granted yourself time to engage mindfully with your breathing and with your body, it may be helpful to allow your heart to remain open to this practice. Allowing your senses to awaken, you may be inclined to open your windows and take in the sounds of nature, or you may choose to play music that supports the flow of your creative nature. With the vision board supplies in proximity, you're ready to begin this activity. You can choose to be completely open as you turn through the pages of your magazines and catalogs. You're not looking for anything in particular—no specific images or words. You're completely open to what attracts your attention without overthinking or being dismissive. When an object on a page resonates with you, simply start cutting it out with mindful attention and purposefulness. Placing each item that you cut on your board, positioning the item in a place that feels most natural to you—but not waiting to arrange the pictures after you've collected them all. Arrange the photos as you encounter them one by one, remembering to breathe, remembering to smile, turning the pages, connecting with what attracts you, cutting and pasting until you feel moved to stop.

Vision Board #2

The steps to completing your second vision board are similar in many ways to the steps for the first. You're invited to begin with mindfulness and openheartedness, and you're also invited to set a specific intention related to creating this board to represent your personal wellness journey. As you flip through the magazines, find items that represent your experiences with stress, the components of the Superwoman Schema, your new coping strategies, your triumphs and challenges with the mindfulness practices described in this book, as well as your engagement in self-compassion. You may not find photos that represent all these topics. It may be ideal to remain open and gentle. You can decide to set a timer (perhaps for forty-five minutes or an hour) to find images, or you may remain open to concluding in a way that feels more natural to you. Instead of placing the images you find on the board in the order that you find them, gather the images in arrangements that feel logical to you or that represent where you want to continue going on your wellness journey, then arrange and attach them to your board as a final step. It's quite possible that you'll find more images than can be pasted on one board, so you may want to have additional blank boards on hand. At your own pace, spend time identifying images that resonate with you, and mindfully select and attach these images until you're ready to end this process.

There are so many additional questions and insights that can come from your mindful vision board experiences. You can even create additional boards with new specific questions or guidelines based on the particular aspects of your health and wellness that you'd like to place in focus. This vision board activity provides you with the opportunity to spend mindful presence with your own experiences, your likes and dislikes, your passions, and your goals in ways that become captured by what you create. Of course, you can also create vision boards that specifically reflect the next steps of your journey, with photographic illustrations of your goals, affirmations, and intentions—including qualities you want to continue to cultivate in yourself, your relationships, and your health. You can frame your vision boards or photograph them to hold on to these revelations. You can even take time to journal what comes up for you from these experiences.

Time for Reflection

Once you've completed your vision boards, set them in a place that allows you to comfortably view and reflect on them—perhaps a large table or counter or on the floor. With mindful presence, notice the similarities and differences of the images and arrangement of images on your boards.

→ What themes arise for you from your first board?

→ Are there any surprises or insights?

→ Does your board help you learn something about yourself, your experiences, or your goals that wasn't as apparent to you before you completed the board?

→ Do the images on the board confirm things you already knew about yourself?

→ How might you grow or move differently in your future based on what you see?

→ What encouragement or inspiration does your board have to offer?

→ Does your board provide information on new goals you can focus on or additional ways you want to continue to change?

→ Reflecting on your second vision board where you were more focused on your personal wellness journey, what revelations or insights are you having?

→ What themes arise?

> → What goals have you achieved and what is there yet to do?
>
> → Spend a little more time with each vision board. What is going on in the images?
>
> → What more can you find?
>
> → What more is there for you to learn?

Conclusion

You have the opportunity to continue to establish new traditions that resonate most with you. You can continue to modify the mindfulness practices you learned in this book. You can continue to reflect upon the principles of the Superwoman Schema and self-care, as you intentionally witness how you grow and transform. You now have tools to create a life of joy and wellness—mindfully and with self-compassion.

Kudos to you for taking time to prioritize your health and wellness. You've learned strategies for overcoming stress and for being your best self. With each step along your path, enjoy the gifts of your ongoing journey. This is only the beginning of a beautiful process.

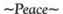

~Peace~

Acknowledgments

Words cannot ever express my gratitude to the New Harbinger staff for recognizing the potential value of this work. Tesilya and team, thank you so much for your gentle and effective guidance. Yvonne Perry! What can I say? You're a true blessing from God! Thank you to my family, friends, mentors, colleagues, prayer warriors, and guardian angels for contributing to my ability to complete this book.

I would like to specifically acknowledge my parents, Dr. Robert Woods and Mrs. Cynthia Diane Hawkins Woods, for consistently being my heroes. Thank you for loving me unconditionally. Thank you to my sister Sonja for being my first role model. I love you more than you know. To my grandparents, aunts, uncles, and cousins: you uplift me in ways that are indescribable.

To my dissertation advisor, Marci Lobel: thank you for supporting me to walk my own path and for believing in my initial ideas about the Superwoman Schema concept. To Dr. Susan Gaylord, Dr. Keturah Faurot, and the entire Harmony and Giscombe Health, Equity, and Arts Lab team—the journey with you has been awesome. I look forward to many years of collaboration and to cheering you on as you continue on your blessed path.

To my students and mentees, I've learned more from you than you've learned from me. I salute you. To my mentorship queens, Dr. Afaf Meleis, Dr. Faye Gary, Dr. Jacquelyn Campbell, Dr. Beverly Malone, Dr. Janice Brewington, Dr. Sylvia Sloan Black, Dr. Vera Moura, and Dr. Giselle Corbie-Smith: your incredible resilience and examples of generosity, strength, and love are dwarfed only by how consistently you let me know how much you believe in me and my abilities. I'm forever grateful. Dr. Clifton Woods III, thank you for your professional guidance and for taking the time to impart wisdom from your experiences in academia.

To the people who live under the same roof as I do—my husband, Kessonga, and my daughters, Zuri and Zola—you make life so much fun! Thank you for the laughter, the hugs, and everything you do to bring joy to my life. Kessonga, thank you for your endless love and support. I love you always. Girls, I'm so proud of you. Please always know how much *you* inspire *me*.

This book is dedicated to the vision and life's work of Dr. Sharon Elliott-Bynum and Dr. Norman B. Anderson. Teamwork makes the dream work! I will always be thankful for the time that I had to learn from your wise excellence.

Finally, to the readers of this book: May you forever find peace and love. Even in the midst of the realities of stressful surroundings, joy is forever present—remember to breathe and remember to smile. Most of all, take care of yourself. The world needs you and your brilliance to be happy and whole.

APPENDIX

Adinkra Symbols and Their Meanings

Studying abroad during the summer between my freshman and sophomore year in college, I had an opportunity to travel to Ghana, West Africa. While there, I became familiar with Adinkra symbols, which were created by people from the Akan region of Ghana. Adinkra symbols are significant components of the Akan culture and are incorporated into architecture, fabrics, and pottery. Each symbol has a distinct meaning related to traditional wisdom about life and nature. Since my first introduction to Adinkra symbols, they have resonated deeply with me, and I find them especially appropriate for illustrating concepts associated with the chapters of this book.

Introduction		**Sankofa** Wisdom, learning from the past to build the future
Chapter 1		**Denkyem** Adaptability
Chapter 2		**Dwennimmen** Strength, humility, wisdom, learning
Chapter 3		**Eban** Love, safety, security
Chapter 4		**Ananse Ntentan** Wisdom, creativity
Chapter 5		**Akoben** Vigilance

Chapter 6		**Nkotim** Loyalty, readiness to serve
Chapter 7		**Akoma** Patience, tolerance
Chapter 8		**Asase Ye Duru** Divinity, providence, power of Mother Earth
Chapter 9		**Bese Saka** Affluence, abundance, unity
Chapter 10		**Aya** Endurance, resourcefulness

Additional Resources

Brondolo, E., K. Byer, P. J. Gianaros, C. Liu, A. Prather, K. Thomas, and C. L. Woods-Giscombé. 2017. *Stress and Health Disparities: Contexts, Mechanisms and Interventions Among Racial/Ethnic Minority and Low Socioeconomic Status Populations: An Official Report of the American Psychological Association.* Washington, DC: APA. https://www.apa .org/pi/health-equity/resources/stress-report.

Magee, R. V. 2019. *The Inner Work of Racial Justice: Healing Ourselves and Transforming Our Communities Through Mindfulness.* New York: TargerPerigee.

Woods-Giscombé, C. L., and A. R. Black. 2010. "Mind-Body Interventions to Reduce Risk for Health Disparities Related to Stress and Strength Among African American Women: The Potential of Mindfulness-Based Stress Reduction, Loving-Kindness, and the NTU Therapeutic Framework." *Complementary Health Practice Review* 15(3): 115–31. doi:10.1177/1533210110386776.

Woods-Giscombé, C. L., and M. Lobel. 2008. "Race and Gender Matter: A Multidimensional Approach to Conceptualizing and Measuring Stress in African American Women." *Cultural Diversity & Ethnic Minority Psychology* 14(3): 173–82. doi:10.1037/1099-9809.14.3.173.

Woods-Giscombé, C. L., M. Lobel, C. Zimmer, C. Wiley Cené, and G. Corbie-Smith. 2015. "Whose Stress Is Making Me Sick? Network-Stress and Emotional Distress in African American Women." *Issues in Mental Health Nursing* 36(9): 710–17. doi:10.3109/01612840 .2015.1011759.

References

Bögels, S. M., and K. Restifo. 2014. *Mindful Parenting: A Guide for Mental Health Practitioners.* New York: Springer.

Carson, J. W., F. J. Keefe, T. R. Lynch, K. M. Carson, V. Goli, A. M. Fras, and S. R. Thorp. 2005. "Loving-Kindness Meditation for Chronic Low Back Pain: Results from a Pilot Trial." *Journal of Holistic Nursing* 23(3): 287–304. doi:10.1177/0898010105277651.

Fredrickson, B. L., M. A. Cohn, K. A. Coffey, J. Pek, and S. M. Finkel. 2008. "Open Hearts Build Lives: Positive Emotions, Induced Through Loving-Kindness Meditation, Build Consequential Personal Resources." *Journal of Personality and Social Psychology* 95(5): 1045–62. doi:10.1037/a0013262.

Gaufberg, E., and R. Williams. 2011. "Reflection in a Museum Setting: The Personal Responses Tour." *Journal of Graduate Medical Education* 3(4): 546–549. doi:10.4300/JGME-D-11-00036.1.

Hutcherson, C. A., E. M. Seppala, and J. J. Gross. 2008. "Loving-Kindness Meditation Increases Social Connectedness." *Emotion* 8(5): 720–24. doi:10.1037/a0013237.

Kabat-Zinn, J. 2013. *Full Catastrophe Living: Using the Wisdom of Your Body and Mind to Face Stress, Pain, and Illness.* New York: Bantam Books.

Lobel, M., C. Dunkel-Schetter, and S. C. Scrimshaw. 1992. "Prenatal Maternal Stress and Prematurity: A Prospective Study of Socioeconomically Disadvantaged Women." *Health Psychology* 11(1): 32–40. doi:10.1037/0278-6133.11.1.32.

Myers, L. J. 1988 *Understanding an Afrocentric World View: Introduction to an Optimal Psychology.* Dubuque, IA: Kendall/Hunt.

Salzberg, S. 1995. *Loving-Kindness: The Revolutionary Art of Happiness.* Boston, MA: Shambhala.

Slavin, R., R. Williams, and C. Zimmermann. 2023. *Activating the Art Museum: Designing Experiences for the Health Professions.* Lanham, MD: Rowman and Littlefield.

Vinesett, A. L., R. R. Whaley, C. Woods-Giscombe, P. Dennis, M. Johnson, Y. Li, P. Mounzeo, M. Baegne, and K. H. Wilson. 2017. "Modified African Ngoma Healing Ceremony for Stress Reduction: A Pilot Study." *The Journal of Alternative and Complementary Medicine* 23(10): 800–04. doi:10.1089/acm.2016.0410.

Williams, R., and C. Zimmermann. 2020. "Twelve Tips for Starting a Collaboration with an Art Museum." *Journal of Medical Humanities* 41(4): 597–601. doi:10.1007/s10912-020-09655-1.

Woods-Giscombé, C. L. 2010. "Superwoman Schema: African American Women's Views on Stress, Strength, and Health." *Qualitative Health Research* 20(5): 668–83. doi:10.1177/1049732310361892.

Woods-Giscombe, C. L., A. M. Allen, A. R. Black, T. C. Steed, Y. Li, and C. Lackey. 2019. "The Giscombe Superwoman Schema Questionnaire: Psychometric Properties and Associations with Mental Health and Health Behaviors in African American Women." *Issues in Mental Health Nursing* 40(8): 672–81. doi:10.1080/01612840 .2019.1584654.

Woods-Giscombé, C. L., D. Carthron, M. Robinson, S. Devane-Johnson, and G. Corbie-Smith. 2016. "Superwoman Schema, Stigma, Spirituality, and Culturally Sensitive Providers: Factors Influencing African-American Women's Use of Mental Health Services." *Journal of Best Practices in Health Professions Diversity* 9(1): 1124–44.

Woods-Giscombé, C. L., and S. A. Gaylord. 2014. "The Cultural Relevance of Mindfulness Meditation as a Health Intervention for African Americans." *Journal of Holistic Nursing* 32(3): 147–60. doi:10.1177/0898010113519010.

Woods-Giscombé, C. L., S. A. Gaylord, Y. Li, C. E. Brintz, S. I. Bangdiwala, J. B. Buse, J. D. Mann, et al. 2019. "A Mixed-Methods, Randomized Clinical Trial to Examine Feasibility of a Mindfulness-Based Stress Management and Diabetes Risk Reduction Intervention for African Americans with Prediabetes." *Evidence-Based Complementary & Alternative Medicine (ECAM)* August: 1–16. doi:10.1155/2019/3962623.

Woods-Giscombé, C. L., M. Lobel, C. Zimmer, C. W. Cene, and G. Corbie-Smith. 2016. "Whose Stress Is Making Me Sick? Network-Stress and Emotional Distress in African-American Women." *Issues in Mental Health Nursing* 36(9): 710–17. doi:10.3109/01612840.2015.1011759.

Yenawine, P., and A. Miller. 2014. "Visual Thinking, Images, and Learning in College." *About Campus* 19(4): 2–8. doi:10.1002/abc.21162.

Cheryl L. Woods Giscombé, PhD, RN, is a distinguished professor, psychiatric nurse practitioner, and social and health psychologist. She is a fellow of the American Academy of Nursing, the Academy of Behavioral Medicine, and the Mind & Life Institute. She is also an elected member of the National Academy of Medicine. Giscombé was named a Leader in the Field by the American Psychological Association, and her community-engaged research on mindfulness, mental health, and wellness for Black women has been consistently funded by the National Institutes of Health and other national foundations and health care organizations for the past twenty years.

Foreword writer Rhonda V. Magee is a renowned mindfulness teacher and innovator of mindfulness-based social justice principles, concepts, and practices. She is professor of law at the University of San Francisco.

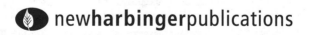

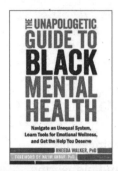
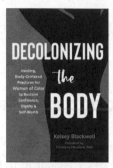
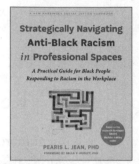
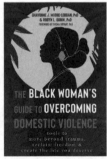
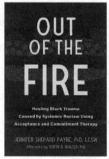
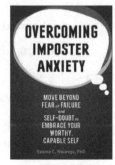